Old and Cold
Hypothermia and Social Policy

Studies in Social Policy and Welfare
Edited by R. A. Pinker

Old and Cold
Hypothermia and Social Policy

Malcolm Wicks

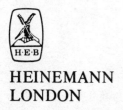

HEINEMANN
LONDON

Published by Heinemann Educational Books Ltd

LONDON EDINBURGH MELBOURNE AUCKLAND
TORONTO HONG KONG SINGAPORE KUALA LUMPUR
NEW DELHI NAIROBI JOHANNESBURG LUSAKA
IBADAN KINGSTON

ISBN 0 435 82939 4
© Malcolm Wicks 1978
First published 1978

Published by Heinemann Educational Books Ltd
48 Charles Street, London WIX 8AH
Typesetting by George Over Ltd, Rugby and London
Printed in Great Britain by
Richard Clay (The Chaucer Press) Ltd, Bungay, Suffolk

Contents

List of Tables in the Text

List of Tables in the Appendix

List of Figures

Acknowledgements

Due to the scale, its inter-disciplinary nature and the number of bodies co-operating in the work, the successful completion of this project depended on the support, advice, help and goodwill of a very large number of people. Only some of them can be mentioned by name here.

The project was initiated at the Centre for Environmental Studies (CES) by its Director at the time, David Donnison. It was prompted by Dr Geoffrey Taylor whose interest in the problem of hypothermia has done much to stimulate public concern. At the outset the CES depended a great deal on the experience and advice of a number of experts and we are grateful for their help. We would like to thank the governors and staff of the CES for their support and, in particular, Neil Piercey who carried out much of the initial organisation.

The Joseph Rowntree Memorial Trust made a grant to the CES to enable the pilot enquiry to be undertaken. The main financial backing for the project came from the Nuffield Foundation and this generous support made the national survey possible. Smaller grants were made by Shell-Mex and B.P. and the Electricity Council.

The project was jointly planned and organised by the CES and the Division of Human Physiology of The National Institute for Medical Research (NIMR), with help from the Geriatric Departments of University College Hospital and The Royal Free Hospital. We wish to thank the staff from each of these bodies who were involved in the project. The project's research team comprised Dr R. H. Fox and Patricia Woodward of the NIMR, Professor A. N. Exton-Smith of University College Hospital, Dr Michael Green of The Royal Free Hospital, David Donnison and the author. I am very much indebted to my colleagues in this team for their advice and support over a number of years. While I take responsibility for any of the book's shortcomings and for all opinions expressed, its contents depend a good deal on the work, knowledge and experience of my fellow researchers.

The fieldwork for both the pilot and national surveys was carried out by Opinion Research Centre (ORC). ORC also played a major role in the planning of the project, the editing of completed questionnaires and the analysis of results. Over and above this however, ORC has maintained an interest and enthusiasm for the project which has been a major reason for its successful completion. In particular thanks are due to John Hanvey, Humphrey Taylor and Charlotte Tatton-Brown. We are also indebted to the nurses who interviewed the old people in our sample.

The author prevailed upon a number of colleagues and friends for comments and advice on the draft version of this book. Thanks are due to John Hanvey, David Donnison, Frank Field, Ken Collins, Norman Exton-Smith and officials of the Department of Health and Social Security, the Supplementary Benefits Commission and the Department of the Environment. David Bull, Tony Lynes, Marigold Johnson, Jonathan Seagrave, Ernest Haseler and David Fruin all provided advice on different aspects of the project or commented on individual chapters. The writing-up of the research has been greatly helped by Irene Morrish who prepared the manuscript for publication.

Anthony Hall collaborated with the author in a postal survey of London Social Services Departments and he is the co-author of Chapter 8 of this book. He also advised on other aspects of the project. We would both like to thank those Social Services Departments who co-operated in our enquiry. Margaret Wicks commented comprehensively on the draft of this book, carried out the statistical tests of significance, drew all the figures and constructed the index.

I am particularly indebted to David Donnison. As Director of the CES he set up the project and has since been a constant source of advice, support and encouragement. Having made this work and the book possible, it is a happy coincidence that some of its recommendations are now addressed to David Donnison as Chairman of the Supplementary Benefits Commission.

My major debt — and that of my research colleagues — is to the large number of old people who co-operated in this extensive and demanding survey. In agreeing to take part many expressed a wish that its results would benefit those pensioners who suffer from the cold. Ultimately that must be the only test of this book's value.

Malcolm Wicks
October 1977

Introduction

This book is about hypothermia and the cold conditions in which many old people live. The research project on which this book is based was devised at a time when there was a developing interest in the problem of the 'old and cold'. Since then there has been a great deal of interest and concern every winter about hypothermia and the effects of cold on the elderly. However, this anxiety is often matched by much ignorance. There has been a good deal of emotion and the generation of much rhetoric, but little hard fact and next to no analysis. Thus estimates about the size of the hypothermia problem vary tremendously. At one extreme some commentators produced a figure of 60,000 deaths every winter from hypothermia while, at the other, the official estimate put the figure at only a dozen or so each year. As we show later, both estimates are highly suspect. Similarly no firm evidence existed about the social circumstances that caused low body temperatures and cold conditions. Again many statements were made about this. But, while some put the emphasis on poverty, others stressed the problems of those old people who were socially isolated, while, for some, bad housing was the key factor.

Early in 1970 the Director of the Centre for Environmental Studies, David Donnison, called together a group of doctors, scientists, nutritionists and experts in housing and welfare to consider what research could usefully be undertaken on this question. David Donnison's initiative was prompted by the work of Geoffrey Taylor who has campaigned for many years on this issue and who saw the need for an extensive enquiry. These experts decided that a national survey should be carried out to investigate the incidence of hypothermia and to consider the social, economic, and environmental living conditions of old people.

Although some small studies had previously been carried out, a national survey had not been undertaken on this question. Such a project would need to combine both scientific measures and the questioning of elderly people on a wide range of social and economic matters and would therefore present many methodological difficulties. Nevertheless a national survey was the only way of obtaining the necessary estimates.

At an early stage in our consultations we sought the advice of Norman Exton-Smith, consultant in geriatrics (and now Professor of Geriatric Medicine) at University College Hospital, a leading authority on hypothermia who was chairman of the British Medical Association's Special Committee on this subject. We also met Ronald Fox of the Division of Human Physiology at the National Institute for Medical Research, an expert on thermo-regulation who had developed techniques for the measurement of body temperatures. Both Professor Exton-Smith and Dr Fox became members of the research team. They were joined by Dr Michael Green, consultant in geriatrics at the Royal Free Hospital and Miss Patricia Woodward of the National Institute for Medical Research. The research team, comprising the above, David Donnison and the author, were responsible for organizing and supervising the project and the preliminary analysis of its results. The fieldwork was organized and conducted by Opinion Research Centre, under the supervision of John Hanvey, and ORC also carried out much of the analysis of the survey's findings.

Some of the main results of the national survey have already been presented in a preliminary report.* The project's researchers have also written a number of subsequent articles based, in part, on the survey's results.† A similar survey was also carried out in the London Borough of Camden. This was designed to allow physiological, medical and other follow-up studies to be undertaken. Some of its results have been reported.‡ An earlier account of the results of the postal survey of social services departments reported in Chapter 8 has also appeared.§

In this book, however, many more results are presented and the relationships between body and room temperatures and social and economic conditions are explored in detail.

Later in this book it will be shown that a small but not insubstantial proportion of elderly people are hypothermic during the winter and that

---

* R. H. Fox, Patricia M. Woodward, A. N. Exton-Smith, M. F. Green, D. V. Donnison, M. H. Wicks, 'Body Temperatures in the Elderly: A National Study of Physiological, Social, and Environmental Conditions', *British Medical Journal*, 27 January 1973. Vol, 1, 200–206.

† *See*, for example, Ronald Fox, *Warmth and the Elderly*, Age Concern, 1974; Michael F. Green, *Hypothermia*, Appendix 3, 'Paying for Fuel', National Consumer Council, HMSO, 1976; A. N. Exton-Smith, 'Accidental Hypothermia', *British Medical Journal*, 22 December 1973; Malcolm Wicks, 'Death in a Cold Climate', *Guardian*, 18 February 1974.

‡ R. H. Fox *et al*, op. cit.; R.H. Fox, 'Physiological Aspects, Results of National and Camden Survey', *Symposium on Hypothermia, Heating and the Elderly*, Centre for Environmental Studies, 1975; K. J. Collins, Caroline Dore, A. N. Exton-Smith, R. H. Fox, I. C. Macdonald and Patricia M. Woodward, 'Accidental Hypothermia and impaired temperature homeostasis in the elderly'. *British Medical Journal*, 1977, 1, 353–356; Cecily de Monchaux, *Psychological Factors in Hypothermia of the Elderly*. Report to the Social Science Research Council, July 1974.

§ Anthony Hall and Malcolm Wicks, 'Winning the Cold War for Old People', *Community Care*, 11 June 1975.

many more – some 10 per cent – have inner body temperatures so low that they are 'at risk' of developing hypothermia. Very many more elderly people live in exceedingly cold homes and, indeed, the vast majority of the elderly experience room temperatures that are below recommended levels. Substantial proportions of pensioners feel cold during the winter months and many would prefer warmer conditions. The results of the national survey, then, offer no support to those who are complacent about hypothermia and who tend to dismiss the 'old and cold' problem as a 'pop' issue that will vanish from the public eye and has no real policy consequences. Rather, the evidence presents an extremely grave picture that poses major challenges to politicians, policy-makers, administrators and those working in the health and social services.

An analysis of low body temperatures and cold conditions by social factors shows that it is not possible to point to specific groups of the elderly that include all (or the vast majority) of those at risk from the cold. Rather the old and cold are to be found among younger and older pensioners, in all house types and tenures, among those living alone and those sharing with others, in different income groups and so on. However, certain groups are more at risk than others. Our results show that the very aged who receive supplementary pensions are much more likely to have low body temperatures than other, younger pensioners. This is probably due to poor health, a declining physiological state and very adverse social conditions.

The results of the national survey strongly suggest that electric blankets are an effective preventative measure in the fight against hypothermia. Old people without electric blankets are more likely to be 'at risk'.

Less than one in four of our sample had central heating, but it was being regularly used and those possessing it had significantly warmer homes than others. However, only one in ten of the elderly heated their bedrooms all night and almost a half did not heat them at all. Most of the elderly found heating expensive and cost was the major reason why those wanting warmer homes did not have them.

It was clear at the outset of our enquiries – and this was confirmed by our results – that a successful attack on the problem of cold conditions would require the marshalling of a number of social policies and services. Indeed the problem has implications not only for the main areas of the welfare state, such as housing, health, welfare and social security, but also for heating systems, fuel-pricing and energy policy. This book presents an analysis of policy and administration in a number of these areas, but does not cover all of them in detail. While some topics, such as supplementary fuel allowances, are discussed comprehensively, several others are noted more briefly. Policy reviews are presented in Chapters 7, 8 and 9.

In the book's concluding chapter it is argued that a four-fold strategy is required to tackle hypothermia and cold conditions. First, there is a need for an identification campaign, involving not only social services but also relatives, neighbours and others who regularly call on the old. Secondly, a number of short-term measures should be undertaken that would have a direct impact on the problem of the old and cold. These include wider and more determined publicity for supplementary benefit heating additions and the launching of a programme to insulate the homes of the old. Thirdly, existing piecemeal arrangements must be replaced by a coordinated and comprehensive approach at both local and national levels. Finally and most importantly, several mainstream social policies must be improved. In particular, better housing and higher pensions are the key to a successful attack on the problem of the old and cold.

Before presenting the results of the national survey and the reviews of policy, the book starts with three background chapters. These discuss the available evidence about the incidence of hypothermia and the nature and effects of the condition, review the social circumstances of Britain's elderly and describe the survey's methodology.

Background

Chapter One: Hypothermia

What is hypothermia? What are its causes? How likely is it to lead to death? How large a problem is it? In this first chapter we will consider these and other questions. It starts by reviewing the development of interest in hypothermia and then analyses the results of surveys conducted into the incidence of this condition. The main aim is to present an introduction to the subject for the layman. Another purpose is to discuss the evidence about the condition that was available at the time that our enquiries began in order to explain why it was necessary to conduct a national survey. Some more recent evidence is discussed in Chapter 10.

The Development of Interest

Interest in 'accidental' hypothermia has grown steadily in recent years. Some of the earliest attention was focused on new-born babies. In 1955 Dr Trevor Mann, in a letter to the *Lancet*[1] reported on a 'new syndrome' of hypothermia in the new-born. In his experience the syndrome was almost confined 'to babies born at home during the winter months'. Two years later an article by Mann and Elliott reported on 14 cases of 'neonatal cold injury'[2]. It concluded that this was a 'not uncommon disorder with a high mortality. Cases generally arise after home confinements, especially in severely cold weather.' However, most cases reported on since then have concerned the elderly. In 1958 J. R. Rees discussed four cases of hypothermia[3] and, in the same year, Dr Emslie-Smith wrote about a further seven cases[4]. The facts of the latter's cases suggested that 'the condition is very much commoner than is generally supposed.'

This interest was maintained throughout the nineteen-sixties with a number of papers in the medical literature dealing with cases of hypothermia and its clinical associations[5]. In 1962, for example, Prescott *et al.* reported on a number of cases of hypothermia being admitted to one small hospital and commented that: 'This relatively high incidence. . . suggests that the condition is more prevalent than is generally believed, and that many cases passed unrecognised.'

1

The reason for a failure to diagnose hypothermia is often due simply to a failure to use the right kind of thermometer. Geoffrey Taylor has noted how the present type of clinical thermometer was devised in the nineteenth century and he remarks that 'it seems that we have all failed to recognise hypothermia, because the clinical thermometer, for historical and arbitrary reasons, does not record it'[6].

In 1964 a special committee of the British Medical Association produced a memorandum on accidental hypothermia[7] because it was felt that there was 'little awareness of the problem'. The Committee referred to the frequent failure to diagnose the condition.

> Most cases of hypothermia are missed because ordinary clinical thermometers do not record the condition. A standard thermometer which begins to register at 95°F (35°C) is misleading, as the actual temperature may be many degrees below this reading. A thermometer reading from 75°F to 105°F (23.9°C to 40.6°C) brings to light many cases which would have remained undiagnosed, and yet such thermometers are not in common use in general practice or in hospital wards unless there is an awareness of the condition.

What is the incidence of hypothermia? At the present time this question cannot be accurately answered. The British Medical Association memorandum had this to say:

> The incidence of the condition is not generally known – many elderly bed-ridden patients may die in their homes without the condition being diagnosed. We therefore suspect that the incidence is very much higher than is commonly supposed. It is particularly high in people over sixty years, but it must not be overlooked that it can also occur at any age and especially in babies.

Although the incidence of hypothermia was unknown, some local studies were carried out in the sixties and their results can be briefly recorded.

Local surveys

In 1968 B. T. Williams[8] reported on a group of old people in one Inner London borough who were aged 70 and over. They were applicants to the welfare department of the local authority and were interviewed between mid-December 1966 and the end of March 1967. Their oral temperatures were taken using a low-reading clinical thermometer placed sub-lingually and left in position for three minutes. The oral temperatures ranged from 91.4°F to 99°F. Six (5 per cent) were below 95°F. Twenty-one (18 per cent) were below 96°F.

Another survey was carried out in Redbridge and Barking in the January, February and March of 1967[9]. Twenty subjects per month were selected in each borough, making a total of 120, each of whom took part for one calendar month. The method of selecting the old people differed between the two boroughs. In Redbridge the subjects were selected at random from a list provided by the Executive Council of all persons aged 75 years or more in one part of the Borough. The Barking subjects were chosen from people aged 60 or more who were receiving home nursing services. Oral temperatures were recorded by leaving the thermometer under the tongue for five minutes. Any subject with an oral temperature of 95°F or below was classified as hypothermic. On this basis 52 (44 per cent) of the subjects had hypothermic readings on one or more occasions. 11 of the subjects had oral temperatures of 95°F or below on 10 or more occasions. Of the 3,275 body temperatures that were taken, 373 (11.4 per cent) were 95°F or below. In Redbridge, 19.3 per cent of the temperatures were at or below this level, and in Barking 3.7 per cent.

A further study, in Hertfordshire during the winters of 1966-7 and 1967-8, was designed to measure the incidence of accidental hypothermia by collecting notifications of admission of cases resident in Hertfordshire to hospitals serving the county[10]. General practitioners were also asked to notify all cases occurring between December 1967 and 31 March 1968. Twenty-five cases of accidental hypothermia were reported, 15 of which were fatal.

The Royal College of Physicians' Survey

The largest survey into hypothermia carried out prior to our own enquiry was by the Royal College of Physicians[11]. This was a survey of the body temperatures of all patients admitted to selected departments of chosen hospitals during the period 1 February to 30 April 1965. The hospitals were asked to take the oral temperatures of all admissions. In those patients in whom the usual clinical thermometer recorded a temperature below 35°C (95°F) the hospitals were asked to use a low-reading thermometer retained in situ for five minutes. For the purposes of this survey a hypothermic patient was defined as one in whom the rectal temperature was below 35°C (95°F).

There were 126 patients found to be admitted with hypothermia – an incidence of 0.68 per cent of all admissions. The Report concludes: 'If this were representative of all hospital admissions in the country during the same three months... there could have been about 9,000 patients admitted to hospitals with temperatures below 35°C (95°F) in the three month period.' The incidence of hypothermia fell from 9.2 per thousand admissions during February to 4.0 per thousand in April. During the coldest week of the survey, with a mean minimum environmental temperature of minus 4.0°C, 19 hypothermic patients were admitted, the highest number for any one week. Infants under 12 months and those aged 75 and above were the two groups with the highest hypothermic admission rates. Infants under 12 months accounted for 1.98 per cent of total admissions, but 23.8 per cent of all hypothermic admissions. Those aged 75 and over made up 11.25 per cent of total admissions, but 28.6 per cent of total hypothermic admissions. Altogether, out of the 126 patients with temperatures below 95°F, 47 died. The Report concluded that ' . . . hypothermia in hospital admissions is common and is associated with a high mortality.' Consequently 'The finding of hypothermia whether in association with extensive disease or as a sole clinical sign is of grave import.' The Report also noted that 'The only clear aetiological association was with environmental temperature, as might be expected, although there was little doubt that social factors also played a part.'

In the years since 1966 when the Royal College's Report was published, public interest in hypothermia, particularly among the elderly, has grown. Dr Geoffrey Taylor who has written many articles about hypothermia has estimated that 'each year between one and five old people in communities of 2,500 die from diseases associated with hypothermia. If this figure is measured against a population of 50 million, it indicates a death rate from hypothermia each winter in Britain of between 20,000 and 100,000'[12].

The press has also become considerably interested in this question and a figure of 60,000 old people dying from hypothermia is frequently quoted. This figure, however, is based on the average difference between the number of deaths in the six winter months and the number of all deaths in the six summer months of the year. As an estimate of the number of old people (or any other group) who die from hypothermia it is completely without foundation. We simply do not know how many people die every year from hypothermia. Regarding the numbers with low body temperatures, the Royal College's study provides some indication. As stated, it projected an estimate of 9,000 patients admitted to hospitals with rectal temperatures below 95°F. This figure is certainly an underestimate of the incidence, however, for two main reasons. Firstly, the survey was carried out in February, March and April, and the 9,000 estimate was for this period. Thus it excluded several of the coldest months, while including April, a spring month. Secondly, it is an estimate of hospital cases and excludes those suffering from hypothermia in their own homes. The local surveys described above show that old people living in their own homes do suffer from low body temperatures. There is evidence that deaths from hypothermia do occur outside of hospitals. A study in Scotland of cases where hypothermia or malnutrition was mentioned on death certificates showed that while 68 per cent had died in hospital, 26 per cent died at home and 6 per cent elsewhere[13].

Social surveys

Apart from the studies that we have mentioned that focused on the medical aspects of hypothermia some other reports have appeared that drew attention to the social aspects of the condition. These were prompted by the concern of those whose community or voluntary work brought them into contact with the elderly.

In 1969 a study was carried out in Birmingham and information was collected on body temperatures (but without using a low-reading thermometer), room temperatures and social conditions. The study found evidence of low room temperatures (40 per cent of those in modern flats and all of those in sub-standard houses had living room temperatures below 60°F) and reported on problems of social isolation, lack of knowledge about benefit entitlement and an unwillingness to use under-floor central heating. The authors of the report called for a more comprehensive survey of hypothermia[14].

When our own project was under way, a similar study to the Birmingham one was undertaken by Task Force in Islington. This survey, carried out in January–April 1971, was conceived 'as a means of obtaining financial help for old people' and paid particular attention to supplementary benefit heating additions. The old people in the survey were already being helped by Task Force and the majority of them had home help and meals-on-wheels.

The study found that many old people were cold at night and that some reported being cold both day and night. Perhaps the most interesting aspect of this study was the fact that, on the basis of its results, 23 requests for equipment and/or fuel grants were sent to the Department of Health and Social Security. Fewer than half of these resulted in an increase in income[15].

What is Hypothermia?

Hypothermia means low body temperature. Sometimes for medical reasons – in surgery for example – hypothermia is induced. For this reason doctors often refer to the condition with which this research is concerned as 'accidental' hypothermia. This is not the place – nor is the author qualified to do so – to discuss in detail the physiological reasons for hypothermia or its medical consequences. However, it will be useful to describe in very elementary terms the human body's thermo-regulatory system, why temperatures can fall and the effects of this.

Thermo-regulation

Some animals have body temperatures which vary with that of the environment and are called poikilothermic (or cold-blooded). Others, including man, are homeothermic, that is, they are usually able to maintain a relatively constant body temperature despite varying external thermal conditions. How is a normal body temperature maintained? From the outset we need to distinguish different types of body temperature, for at any one time there is no one, single body temperature. Temperatures will vary from one part of the body to another and one can distinguish between temperatures on the body surface and those of the inner body or 'core'. And temperatures will also vary from one part of the body surface to another and also within the core. In fact medical practitioners and scientists are able to measure temperatures in a number of different places: the mouth temperature (measured sub-lingually) and the rectal temperature are common in medical practice. Skin temperatures can also be recorded and, as is described in Chapter 3, the temperature of urine was measured for this survey.

The most important temperatures to maintain at an adequate level are those of the deep body or core. In simple terms, while it is not too serious for the mouth temperature to drop some degrees below 'normal', it is, at least potentially, a very serious matter if there is a significant drop in the temperature of the inner body. In fact the body has various means of maintaining deep body temperature homeostasis − i.e. maintaining it at a reasonable or normal level. These defence mechanisms strive to protect the body against both cold and hot environments. When these are working adequately deep body temperature homeostasis is maintained despite adverse thermal conditions.

Ronald Fox has said that:—

> In engineering terms we can describe the thermo-regulatory system as a closed-loop negative feed-back control system with a built-in 'set point' and temperature sensors[16].

He has described how the skin can be seen as:—

> The barrier between the physiology of the body on the one hand and the environment on the other, and the system is emphasised as a controlled heat loss system in which the metabolic heat produced by the internal organs is trans-

ported by the blood stream to the skin where it is lost into the environment; the rate at which the heat is transported being controlled to maintain the temperature in the deeper parts of the body close to 37°C. The heat is transported in the blood stream through the vessels going from the interior of the body to the skin surface and back again, thus by increasing the amount of blood passing through the skin, which we call cutaneous vasodilation, the amount of heat transported is increased; whereas by reducing the amount of blood flowing through the skin vessels, or cutaneous vasoconstriction, the amount of heat transported to the skin and lost to the environment is decreased[17].

Temperatures are regulated by the hypothalamus in the brain. Fox has described how this works:—

There is a hypothalamic control centre in the central nervous system which acts rather like a computer. It receives signals as inputs from temperature receptors situated in the skin which are of two types, cold and warm receptors; there are also known to be deep receptors in the interior of the body and the hypothalamic centre itself is believed to be sensitive to changes in temperature. These sensory inputs provide information to the centre on the temperature status of the individual. In some way, which we do not fully understand, they are compared with an absolute temperature reference, so that we have a 'set point' mechanism, in other words, the centre is able to determine whether action should be taken to get rid of more heat to bring the temperature back to the 'set point' or whether it should reduce the rate of heat loss to bring the temperature up to the 'set point'. To achieve this adjustment there are effectors or outputs from the hypothalamic controller which run to the structures in the skin responsible for temperature regulation. The most important of these are the blood vessels, but there are also nerves which run to sweat glands and to the piloerecti muscles which cause goose-pimples[18].

It is in this way that the human body is able to maintain its body temperature homeostasis. However, in extreme thermal conditions this system will be unable to cope and in such circumstances two defence mechanisms are available – sweating in hot conditions and shivering in cold conditions.

Causes of hypothermia

Hypothermia can be the result of exogenous factors (i.e. adverse thermal conditions – the cold) or endogenous or internal factors. The first category includes, for example, exposure on mountains and in the sea. However, it is the cold conditions in the homes of the elderly with which this book is concerned. The second category includes a range of illnesses and conditions, as well as the effects of certain drugs and alcohol. The British Medical Association memorandum stated:—

Clinical disturbances which may predispose to hypothermia include:
(1) endocrine conditions (myxoedema and hypopituitarism);
(2) neurological disorders (falls and drop attacks, cerebrovascular accidents, paraplegia, head injuries);
(3) mental inpairment and confusional states;
(4) conditions causing vascular collapse, especially myocardial infarction;
(5) severe infections, especially pneumonia; and
(6) drugs affecting the temperature regulation of the body (chlorpromazine and other phenothiazine tranquillizers, barbiturates, and alcohol)[19].

Relationship between endogenous and exogenous factors

The distinction between endogenous and exogenous causes of hypothermia is an important one. However, both factors may be important in some cases. To take one specific category, it would seem likely that some of those living rough, out-of-doors in winter put themselves at greater risk of hypothermia by drinking too much alcohol[20]. More common – and directly relevant to this study – will be cases of elderly people who live in cold accommodation suffering from one or more medical conditions which may have a temperature-reducing effect.

Green notes that: 'Hypothermia may arise as the primary disease in an old person or it may arise concurrently with or follow other diseases, but in all these situations it is regarded as a damaging disorder in its own right, causing illness or even death[21]'. He gives an example: 'a confused, partially sighted old lady wanders out to the outside W.C. at night, falls because of an abnormally low blood pressure, breaks her leg and succumbs to hypothermia because she was already cold from living in poverty and a cold flat and also suffering from defective temperature control reflexes[22]'.

The evidence is not available to distinguish the relative importance of each of these two causes of hypothermia. The special BMA Committee felt that in most cases causes are mixed and that in the elderly 'both factors seem to be involved in varying proportions.' However, it was the Committee's view that 'exposure to cold seems to be the overriding cause[23].' In Chapter 4 we discuss how the existence of endogenous hypothermia 'confuses', to some extent, the analysis of the results of a national survey designed primarily to consider the effects of exogenous factors on body temperature.

How low is too low?

Hypothermia means low body temperature. But what is meant by 'low'? At what level can hypothermia be said to exist? The generally accepted cut-off point is 35°C or 95°F. Thus the Royal College of Physicians' report refers to 'those with rectal temperatures below 35°C (95°F)[24].'

Clearly, however, such a definition is arbitrary and one needs to be extremely cautious about interpreting the significance of those classified as hypothermics and those not (for example, someone with a deep body temperature of, say, 35.1°C). It is partly for this reason that, for the analysis of the results of our national survey, we defined those with temperatures below 35.5°C (95.9°F) as being 'at risk' of developing hypothermia. But what does it mean to be hypothermic in medical terms? Does it necessarily mean that the person is ill? And what is the risk of death? In fact there are no straightforward answers to these questions.

What do we know about the mortality rate of hypothermics? In the Royal College survey 37% of the 126 hypothermic hospital admissions died. Divided into temperature categories 73% of those below 30°C died, 33% of those between 30°C – 32.9°C and 32% between 33.0°C – 34.9°C. It is important to remember that these included all age groups and that in most cases other diseases were present. However, there were 17 patients in whom hypothermia was the principal diagnosis made by the hospital. Of these 10 were aged 65 and over and 5 of these died[25].

The Royal College's evidence, and that from other hospital cases, therefore shows that hypothermia is associated with a high mortality rate, but that this is particularly the case at very low temperature levels.* However, death can occur at higher temperatures than these and much will depend on the existence of other diseases and their effect on, and their relationship to, low core temperatures.

In their memorandum the BMA Committee stated that the clinical aspects of hypothermia could be divided into three fairly distinct phases:—

    (1) Initial response to cold (98.4° – 90°F; 36.9° – 32.2°C) is vasoconstriction of the skin arterioles; this is accompanied by increase in pulse rate in the early

---

*The initial temperatures of the 5 elderly persons (referred to above) in the Royal College study who died, where hypothermia was the principal diagnosis, were 83.0°F; 81.6°F; 'below 85.0°F'; 76.2°F and 80.0°F.

stages and by diuresis. The normal protective mechanism of shivering is often absent in old people. The patients do not necessarily complain of cold.

(2) At a body temperature below 90°F (32.2°C) shivering is not observed but muscular rigidity is a striking feature; the skin is pale, cold and dry; oedema is often present, sometimes in the face, simulating myxoedema; mental processes are slow and consciousness is impaired and later lost; blood-pressure is low or unrecordable; respiratory and heart rate may be slow; atrial fibrillation is common with slow, irregular pulse; characteristic ECG changes are often seen.

(3) The more profound is the hypothermia the more serious are the disturbances of function in the vital organs with multiple arterial thrombosis affecting particularly the heart, intestines and pancreas, and the more likely is a fatal outcome.

The history is almost always one of progressive confusion; slowing speech, ataxia, and involuntary movements are common. The patient's responses are slow. Hypothermic elderly people do not necessarily look ill, but the skin is pale or cyanosed and sometimes has a puffy consistency. Those parts of the body which are normally protected feel cold to the touch, and the most valuable diagnostic measure is to place the hand on the patient's abdomen. The disturbance of consciousness is related to the degree of hypothermia[26].

The BMA Committee also stated that the following complications may occur in hypothermic patients:

(1) bronchopneumonia;
(2) haemorrhagic phenomena such as gastric erosions and acute pancreatitis;
(3) multiple-visceral necroses and myocardial infarction; and
(4) gangrene of limbs due to the intense peripheral vasoconstriction[27].

Conclusion

Hypothermia means low body temperature, but much depends on what body temperature is measured. In our discussion we placed particular emphasis on the critical importance of measuring the inner body or core temperature. The generally accepted cut-off point in the diagnosis of hypothermia is 35°C or 95°F, but this is clearly arbitrary and there is a need for some caution in the classification of hypothermia. Undoubtedly hypothermia is a very dangerous condition. It has a high mortality rate and this is particularly the case at very low temperature levels. Hypothermia is also associated as both cause and effect with other illnesses.

Our brief review of the medical literature on hypothermia indicates a growing interest in this condition over the last fifteen years. Small local surveys and the larger Royal College survey show that the incidence of hypothermia might be higher than many have thought in the past. Local surveys focusing on the social aspects of the problem of the old and cold have also been undertaken. These have found evidence of cold conditions and other social problems and much unmet need. On the basis of these studies, however, it is impossible to make reliable estimates of incidence. What is the distribution of inner body temperatures among the elderly population? What proportion of the old have temperatures below the hypothermic level? How many live in cold conditions? The national survey was designed to answer questions such as these.

Background

Chapter 2
The Social Circumstances of Britain's Elderly

This chapter briefly analyses the social and economic circumstances of Britain's elderly population. This will provide a context in which to assess the results of our national survey. Specifically it will point to testable hypotheses about the relationship between temperature levels and the social conditions of old people. The services and benefits that are available to elderly people and which directly relate to the problems of the old and cold will be considered. Whether or not those 'at risk' from the cold are receiving these services and benefits will be considered in later chapters and the policy implications of these findings will be discussed in the conclusion to this book.

Demography and Household Composition

This century has witnessed an 'ageing' of the population. Thus, while the United Kingdom's total population increased from just over 38 millions in 1901 to approaching 56 millions in 1971, the numbers over retirement age increased from 2.4 millions to 9.1 millions during the same period. As Table 2.1 shows, the retirement age groups as a percentage of the population rose from 6.2% to 16% during this seventy-year period and the estimates for 2001 show a similar position.

Table 2.1

Elderly Population, U.K. 1901 – 2001
(Millions)

	1901	1931	1971	2001
Men (65+)	0.8	1.4	2.8	3.2
Women (60+)	1.6	2.9	6.3	6.3
Total	2.4	4.3	9.1	9.5
Total population	38.2	46.0	55.7	58.3
Retired as % of total population	6.2	9.6	16.0	16.3

Source: Based on Table 1.1, *Social Trends*, No. 7, 1976. Projections for year 2001 are 1975-based.

This 'ageing' of the population, due to the combination of a decline in birth rates and an increase in life expectancy, has led to a certain amount of gloomy forecasting about its effect on the social and economic life of the nation. It is paradoxical that this welcome phenomenon has been so heralded. As Titmuss has noted: 'Viewed historically, it is difficult to understand why the gradual emergence in Britain of a more balanced age structure should be regarded as a "problem of ageing".[1]' Titmuss reminds us that this should be regarded as a matter for satisfaction. Yet while they are not themselves a problem, certain 'problems' do affect the elderly or, more precisely, certain groups of them. One of the inevitable consequences of an 'ageing' population is that, compared with the past, a greater proportion of the elderly are now 'very aged'.

In 1901 1.1% of all males and 1.5% of all females were aged 75 years and over. By 1971 the proportions were 3% and 6.3% respectively. In absolute terms the numbers aged 75 and over were some five times greater in 1971 than at the turn of the century, an increase from 0.5 million in 1901 to 2.6 million in 1971[2]. It is estimated that the numbers aged 75 years and over in England will increase by nearly a third by 1995 rising to just under 3 million. The number aged 85 years and over is expected to increase by over 50% by 1995, rising from 448,000 (in 1976) to 692,000[3].

Large numbers of those reaching retirement age can expect to live quite a while longer. In fact, in 1971, a man (aged 65) could look forward to an average life expectancy of 12 years, while a woman (aged 60) had an average life expectancy of 19.7 years[4]. As more and more people expect to survive into their eighties and nineties, concern has increasingly focused on the very aged as a vulnerable group among the elderly generally and their social circumstances will be specifically looked at in this chapter. When presenting the results of our national survey we will consider whether the very aged are more likely to have low body temperatures than younger pensioners.

It is well known that more women than men survive into old age. In 1975 there were approximately 6,483,000 women aged 60 and over compared to 4,520,000 men. This sex-differential increases with age: 72% of those aged 80 or over were female[5].

It follows from this differential survival pattern and also from the tendency for women to marry at a younger age than men, that the marital status of Britain's elderly varies significantly according to sex. A married woman is very likely to outlive her spouse and consequently the proportion of widows among the female population will increase with age. Thus, whereas in 1971 22% of females aged 60-64 were widows, the figure was over 58% for the 75-79 age group, rising to 76% for those aged 85 or over. The pattern for men is very different: only 10% of those aged 65-69 are widowed and even for those aged 80-84 the figure is only 40%[6].

One noticeable feature about the social circumstances of the elderly is the large proportion who live alone, and this proportion has been steadily rising in recent decades: in 1951 13.4% of people of pensionable age lived alone, the figure was 19.5% in 1961 and by 1971 had risen to 24.2%[7]. Since the last Census the proportion seems to have increased. The General Household Survey figures for those aged 65 and over are 30.1%, 1972; 30.6%, 1973 and 32.8%, 1974[8].

Again the pattern changes with increasing age. Whereas in 1974, only 17% of household members aged 60-64 lived alone, 42% of those aged over 80 did so[9]. The pattern varies in other ways too. As the General Household Survey Introductory Report comments:

> Among persons aged 80 or over, there was a decline in the proportion living with another adult and a corresponding increase in the proportion living either with two other adults or in households containing children. This is because old people, faced by widowhood and a decline in self-sufficiency, often return to live with their children and their children's families[10].

It would be wrong to conclude hastily that an old person living alone definitely constitutes a 'problem'. Often this will be far from true. Many spinsters will have lived alone for a number of years; so, too, will have many widows. Large numbers in these groups have adjusted well to living on their own and will cherish their independence. Those living alone are by no means necessarily 'socially isolated'. We were nevertheless interested to analyse body and room temperatures by household composition to see if those living alone were more likely to be 'at risk'. In one sense this group do face definite risks. As Exton-Smith observes: 'A common story is of an old person who falls after attempting to get out of bed at night; he remains on the floor for several hours, often partly clad, and is discovered only the next day by a neighbour or a home help'[11]. Some of those living on their own clearly face the danger of not being found for some time and, in some tragic cases, death comes before help.

It is, however, reasonable to expect that it will be the 'socially isolated' elderly, rather than the larger group of those who live alone, who will feature significantly among those likely to be 'at risk' from the cold. Several studies have sought to measure the phenomenon of social isolation[12]. The conclusions of a study in Britain, Denmark and the United States were as follows:—

> Broadly speaking, only a very small minority were found to be living in extreme isolation, in the sense that a week or even a day could pass without human contact. Between 2% and 3% of the elderly in the three countries lived alone,

had had no visitors in the previous week, and had had no human contact on the day previous to interview[13].

The authors of this study found that the isolated are generally persons who are (1) older than average, (2) single or widowed, (3) lacking children and other relatives living nearby, (4) retired from work and infirm. 'It is usually the combination of three or more of these factors rather than any one factor that produces isolation'[14].

Physical Mobility

Increasing physical frailty is an obvious problem to be found among the aged. Old age does not inevitably bring in its train extreme immobility, but a small proportion of the elderly are severely physically restricted. The survey by Shanas, Townsend *et al.* in 1962 found that 3% of Britain's population aged 65 or over were bedfast, while a further 11% were housebound. It is significant that a higher proportion of women than men were bedfast or housebound − 18% as against 7%. While the differential age structure of the sexes partly explains this, it is the case that old men are generally more physically mobile than old women[15].

The relatively immobile might be expected to be among those 'at risk' from the cold. Exton-Smith has explained that immobility can be associated with hypothermia. Patients suffering from certain conditions are often confined to bed and 'the lack of muscular activity leads to inadequate heat production'[16]. To a degree this will also be true for the non-bedfast, but relatively immobile elderly. It is reasonable to assume that much will depend on household circumstances. The old person living with his or her spouse or with children or others will probably be perfectly well cared for and indeed the incapacitated are more likely to be living with others. Nevertheless a significant group of the incapacitated do live alone: the 1962 Survey showed that 25% of those with high incapacity lived alone. These people represented 1% of elderly males and 4% of elderly females[17]. Unless this group received adequate domestic support − either from family or social agencies − they might well be suffering the effects of cold conditions.

Housing

Britain's elderly live in poorer housing than the rest of the population. This section briefly presents evidence in support of this general statement.

Much of the nation's housing stock is old: estimates vary but all show that in 1971 approximately one-third of dwellings were built before

1919[18]. Old people are much more likely to be living in this older accommodation than younger groups. This is to be expected and clearly reflects the fact that many old people have lived in their homes for many years. Old housing is not, as such, a problem for the elderly, but its association with physically inadequate standards is. Old housing is more likely to mean 'unfit' housing or housing that lacks basic amenities. Wroe has summarized the relevant information from the 1971 General Household Survey that shows the distribution of these conditions between different age groups.

Table 2.2

Age of Dwelling and Amenities by Age of Head of Household, Great Britain, 1971

	Age of Head of Household				
	25–44	*65–69*	*70–79*	*80+*	*All 65+*
	%	%	%	%	%
Percentage of households in accommodation:—					
Built before 1919	24	37	39	42	39
Lacking fixed bath	5	14	16	20	16
Lacking internal W.C.	9	19	21	23	20
Without central heating	57	73	77	82	76

Source: D. C. L. Wroe, 'The Elderly', *Social Trends*, No. 4, 1973, H.M.S.O., 1973 (based on General Household Survey data).

Table 2.2 shows that dwellings where the head of the household is aged 65 and over are more likely to be older than those for younger households and are much more likely to lack basic amenities. It also shows that *within* elderly households, the older the household head the more likely it is that dwellings are old and amenities are lacking. Thus of those aged 80 and over 42% live in dwellings built before 1919, 20% lack a fixed bath and 23% are without an internal W.C.

Of particular interest is the evidence about central heating. This shows that younger age groups are more likely to possess central heating, while 76% of all households with heads aged 65 and over lack it. Again the very aged are less likely to have this amenity than younger pensioners. Only 18% of those aged 80 and over have central heating.

The evidence about the relative deprivation of the very aged (among the elderly generally) suggests that it is those old people who live alone who experience some of the worst housing conditions. This is confirmed by evidence from the General Household Survey[19] which shows that in 1973 individuals aged 60 and over were more likely to lack amenities than older small households. And only 25% of individuals aged 60 or over had central heating, compared to 32% of older small households.

Table 2.3

Household Type by Tenure, Great Britain, 1973

	Older Small Households* %	Individuals Aged 60 + %	Total Households %
Owner occupied – owned outright	45	36	22
Owner occupied – with mortgage	6	2	27
Rented with job/business	2	1	4
Rented from local authority/new town	31	36	32
Rented from housing association	1	1	1
Rented privately unfurnished	15	22	11
Rented privately furnished	0	2	3

* i.e. 2 persons aged 16 or over, at least one of whom is aged 60 or over.
Source: General Household Survey 1973, Table 2.1(a).

The tenure distribution of the elderly population (shown in Table 2.3) is different from that of all households and there is also a difference between older small households and individual households where the person is aged 60 and over. Thus older small households, compared to total households, are slightly more likely to be owner-occupiers; about as likely to be council tenants, while more of them are unfurnished private tenants (but very few are furnished tenants). Old people living alone, however, are under-represented among owner-occupiers, are more commonly in the council sector, and are more likely than others to be private tenants.

The general over-representation of both elderly household groups in the privately rented sector is a major reason why the elderly more commonly lack basic amenities than others. Compared to other tenure groups privately rented housing is older and is more likely to be 'unfit for human habitation[20]' or lacking basic amenities[21]. It also seems likely that elderly owner-occupiers live in accommodation that is in worse condition than other dwellings in this sector, firstly because of its greater age,[22] and secondly because of the problems (both financial and those stemming from physical frailty) of many elderly.

The possession of central heating varies considerably according to tenure. In 1973 65% of all owner-occupiers with a mortgage had central heating; 40% of those who owned outright possessed it; 28% of local authority and new town tenants; and only 11% of privately rented unfurnished tenants[23].

A final factor of relevance to our study is the size of the dwellings occupied by the elderly population. Eighty per cent of older smaller households had more bedrooms than the 'bedroom standard' (38% having two or more bedrooms above the standard), and 70% of individuals aged 60 or more had accommodation with a number of bedrooms above the standard (34% with two or more bedrooms above the standard)[24].

While space is generally considered an advantage, housing which is larger than need requires can become a problem for some old people – too many rooms to keep clean, decorated and adequately heated.

Financial Circumstances of the Elderly

Many of Britain's elderly suffer from relative poverty[25]. For most, old age brings with it retirement from employment and consequently an often dramatic decline in living standards. Yet while the average retired person's income will be much lower than that of a working person, there is much variation. The level of income in old age depends on many factors. Previous employment will be a major one: a former salaried employee may well be drawing a private pension and have accumulated substantial savings on which to draw; a manual worker is less likely to be receiving a private pension and, if he is, it will often be small. Health in old age is also important: a fit person may go on working full-time after the normal retirement age or, if retired, may earn through part-time work. The family situation is sometimes influential: a retired person may well derive economic support from a large extended family: children may make regular payments to their parents or meet occasional expenses. Some old persons will live with their children and have their living standards improved in this way. The spinster, on the other hand, may suffer economically from her social isolation.

The nature and extent of poverty in old age will depend to a large degree on the adequacy of state social security. But standards of living will also be crucially affected by whether or not there are additional sources of income available. The last detailed enquiry into income in old age was undertaken in 1965 and published in the report 'Financial and Other Circumstances of Retirement Pensioners'[26]. This Report showed that while most old persons have at least one additional source of income, widowed and single persons are less likely to have such resources than married couples. In part this is due to the fact that compared with the latter, the single and widowed are generally older and additional sources of income decline with age for the reasons mentioned earlier. It is therefore possible to see in what circumstances chronic poverty can occur. The very aged will be less able to work part-time due to physical frailty, most will receive no private pension or, at best, a very small one and savings will vanish all too quickly. If they receive no family support (and sometimes their children will be pensioners themselves) these people will be in desperate poverty. And, as we saw earlier, many of them will also be living alone.

The next group to identify are single women. The 1963 Inquiry found that: 'Proportionately more married couples . . . had additional income, compared with single pensioners, and the proportions without additional incomes of any kind were consistently and conspicuously higher among single women in all age groups than those found among men, whether married or single.' The fact that single women are often poor is due to several factors: women live longer than men and this, together with the differential age of marriage, will mean that many women have to live their last years on their own. In addition a significant proportion of elderly women were never married at all. Women's wages have traditionally been very much lower than men's and so the opportunity for saving is small. Most former women employees would not have been in private pension schemes. And to exacerbate these sexual inequalities, state social security has always treated women harshly.

Importance of state benefits

For the minority of elderly persons with no additional source of income the existence and scope of state social security benefits is all-important. However it is also important for those with an independent source of income and, in the words of Dorothy Wedderburn, the level of benefits is 'crucial in determining the standard of living of the majority of the elderly'[27]. The 1962 Survey showed the percentage of aggregate money income from government income to be 48%, 51% and 71% for couples, single men and single women respectively[28].

The British national insurance system was originally intended to protect all contributors to the scheme against the worst effects of loss of earnings. It was supposed by William Beveridge that any person receiving an insurance pension would, following a 20-year transition period, be automatically above the poverty line – the national assistance and, since 1966, the supplementary benefits level. One of the main reasons for the continuance of poverty in old age is quite simply that insurance pension levels have been consistently below the supplementary benefits standard. For example, in October 1973, the insurance pension for a single person was £7.75, whereas the supplementary benefits level for a single retired person was £8.15 (excluding the 'rent' payment).

The level of national insurance pensions as a proportion of national average earnings has been distinguished over time by its consistency.

Although levels have been increased fairly frequently (and increasingly so in recent times) they have only kept up with average earnings. The exception is the period since July 1974 when increases have represented a real improvement[29]. In general pensions have maintained their real value but this has been low compared to the standards enjoyed by the general population.

Supplementary benefits

For the group of pensioners with no source of income apart from national insurance pensions, as well as for those receiving only a little additional income, supplementary benefits play a critical role. The small proportion of elderly persons who do not receive national insurance pensions are also heavily dependent on supplementary benefits.

Supplementary pensions are a major part of the social security system for the elderly: in December 1976, 1,687,000 people were receiving supplementary pensions, and about 23% of all the retired are supported by them[30]. As would be expected supplementary pensioners are, on average, older than other retired people. Sixteen per cent of those aged 65-69 received supplementary benefit at the end of 1975, compared to 26 per cent of those aged 70-84 and 28 per cent of the over 84 group. Three-quarters of those benefiting from supplementary benefit were women[31].

It is important to note that large numbers of the elderly have incomes low enough to qualify for supplementary benefit but do not, in fact, receive it. Failure to claim benefit may be due to ignorance, the system's complexity, a sense of pride and independence or fear of stigma. An official enquiry in 1965[32] estimated that over 700,000 pensioners did not get the benefits for which they were eligible. The Supplementary Benefits Commission Report for 1975 estimated that of all pensioners eligible for some supplementary pension, 75% were receiving one[33]. Many non-claimants are the poorest elderly who will find it most difficult to keep their homes adequately heated. For this reason a division of the elderly into recipients or non-recipients of benefit is, at best, only a rough approximation of the division between the poor and the not-so-poor elderly.

Expenditure patterns

How do the elderly spend their incomes? And, in particular, what proportion of their expenditure goes on fuel and other basic essentials? The annual Family Expenditure Survey is the best source of information on these questions. Tabel 2.4 shows the proportions of expenditure that go on housing, fuel and food — arguably the three major essentials — and compares the figures for elderly households with all households.

The main point shown up by this table is that, compared to all households, a large proportion of the expenditure of the elderly goes on housing, fuel and food. There is also variation between the different elderly house-

Table 2.4

Expenditure on Commodity or Service
as Percentage of Total Household Expenditure, 1975

	Housing	Fuel	Food	Total Expenditure on Housing Fuel and Food	Other Expenditure
One Adult:					
Men aged 65+	20.7	9.9	26.3	56.9	43.1
Women aged 60+	23.7	10.2	26.4	60.3	39.7
Man and Woman:					
Head aged 65+	16.8	8.3	27.7	52.8	47.2
All Households	13.1	5.5	24.8	43.4	56.6

Source: Family Expenditure Survey 1975, Table 33.

hold types. Due to a high proportionate expenditure on housing, women aged 60 or over who are living alone spend a higher proportion of their money on the three main items than do men living alone, 60.3% compared to 56.9%. Those living alone spend proportionately more on fuel than do married couples. It has been shown that it is the single woman who is generally the poorest among the elderly. The effects of this on expenditure can be seen. In 1975, only 39.7% of total expenditure of women pensioners living alone went on items other than the three main ones. As their average total weekly expenditure was £19.97 this meant that less than £8.74 was spent on such items.

It is useful to see how expenditure patterns vary by income within the elderly community and Table 2.5 shows the situation in 1975 for those aged 65 and over who were living alone. As would be expected the amount available for spending on items other than housing, fuel and food increases with income. The position for the poorest group – those with weekly incomes of £8 and under £15 – is that, while their housing costs are proportionately low, their spending on fuel and food is proportionately high. On average this poorest group had only 34.1% left to spend on items other than the three main ones.

People in this group are among the poorest in Britain. Events that most can take in their stride – the need to buy a new saucepan, shoe-repairs, a worn-out coat – can seriously affect life at the margin. Given that housing costs have to be met, most budgeting will involve food and fuel. If extra warmth is required, during a particularly cold winter spell, less spending on food may often be the inevitable consequence.

Table 2.5

*Expenditure of One-Adult Households aged 65+
as Percentage of Weekly Income*

| | Weekly Income | | | | |
	£8 and under £15	£15 and under £20	£20 and under £30	£30 or more	All House-holds*
Average Total Income (£)	13.06	16.19	22.71	31.29	18.87
Housing	17.3	26.7	22.2	24.9	24.3
Fuel, light and power	14.5	12.1	9.3	7.2	10.7
Food	34.1	30.9	23.6	20.3	27.2
Other	34.1	30.3	44.9	47.6	37.8

* i.e. all the adult households aged 65+
Source: Family Expenditure Survey, 1975, based on Table 6. See this table for details of percentage standard errors.

From this brief review of the available evidence several facts stand out. First and foremost is that, relative to the population as a whole, the elderly are generally poor. This general point needs to be remembered when identifying the groups among the elderly that are the poorest. Certain groups do stand out nevertheless and when considering the survey's findings about temperature levels we will pay particular attention to these.

Poverty is associated with increasing age: often unable to work part-time, lacking any private pension (or possessing only a small one eroded by inflation) and with savings spent, the very aged have particular financial problems. Single and widowed women are the other group that include many of the poorest. Usually without a private pension, they will be worse off than either single male pensioners or married couples. The two groups – the very aged and single and widowed women – do, of course, greatly overlap. It is the older spinster or widow who bears the brunt of poverty in old age.

The poorest among the elderly will be eligible for supplementary benefits and almost a quarter of all pensioners are supported by them. Supplementary pensioners are then, by definition, broadly the poorest old people. There are, however, a large number of elderly people who, though eligible for supplementary benefits, do not claim them.

Health and Welfare Services

The final part of this chapter presents a brief review of some of the health and welfare services that may be available to the elderly. The use of these services was considered in the first General Household Survey and its main findings are presented in Table 2.6.

Table 2.6

Rate per 1,000 using Six Domiciliary Services in a One-Month Reference Period (England and Wales, 1971)

Service	Age	
	65 – 74	75 +
Health Visitor	6.9	16.4
District Nurse	17.1	57.9
Chiropodist	8.1	41.5
Home Help	24.0	97.8
Meals on Wheels	9.8	26.6
Welfare Officer	7.7	17.2
Persons using one or more of these services	56.2	188.6
Persons using none of these services	943.8	811.4

Source: General Household Survey, *Introductory Report*, H.M.S.O., 1973, Table 8.45.

The main finding from this table is that the vast majority of old people do not regularly receive domiciliary services: 94% of those aged 65-74 and 81% of those aged 75 or over were found to be using none of these services in a one-month reference period. The other important point that emerges is that while the elderly in general are much more likely to receive services than other adults (only 1% of those aged 45-65 received services in the one-month period, for example) it is the older pensioners who make most call on these services. Approximately 19% of those aged 75 or over received one or more services during the month, compared to under 6% of those aged 65-74. The table also shows the relative importance of certain services and particularly home helps: almost 10% of those aged 75 or over had a home help during the month.

It is obvious that several of the services listed in Table 2.6 can play a part in the prevention of hypothermia and the more general problem of the cold. But are those most 'at risk' from low temperatures more likely to be receiving these services? This question will be explored in Chapter 6. The policy and administrative implications of our findings for social services departments are discussed in Chapter 8.

Conclusion

Apart from sketching in some of the background against which to view the results presented in later chapters, this analysis of the social circumstances of Britain's elderly has thrown up some specific hypotheses about the causes of hypothermia and cold conditions. The 'ageing' of the population means that many old people will survive into their 80s and 90s. The very aged are generally regarded as more vulnerable than younger pensioners. Are they likely to be more at risk of hypothermia? Most of the very aged are women and a significant proportion are widows. Are they more likely to suffer the effects of the cold? What about the increasing numbers of the elderly who live alone? Are they in particular danger during the winter? Similarly, do the physically immobile suffer particularly from the cold?

Does the type of tenure of housing relate in any specific way to cold conditions? Do those in physically inadequate housing face particular risks? Does central heating produce warmer conditions? Or do worries about expense or a reluctance to use new forms of heating negate its beneficial effects? And what about income? Is it the case (as many have argued) that poverty is the major cause of hypothermia? Are those dependent on supplementary benefits, for example, more likely to be in jeopardy? Finally, how does the Welfare State make an impact on the problem? At the very least, are those in the coldest conditions and those at risk in touch with the health and personal social services? Drawing on the results of our national survey, these questions will be discussed in Chapters 5 and 6.

Background

Chapter 3
Scientific Methods
and Survey Techniques

In Chapter 1 we reviewed the evidence about the incidence and causes of hypothermia. It was shown there that a number of local surveys had been carried out and also a survey of hospital admissions. However, none of these surveys enabled us to make an estimate about the size of the problems of hypothermia or the 'old and cold'. Such estimates could only be made on the basis of a national survey of a large, randomly selected sample of old people. In this chapter we give details of how this survey was organized, but we start by noting the methods that were used to measure temperatures.

Scientific Methods

Body temperatures

In Chapter 1 we stressed the importance of the inner body or core temperature. Accordingly a major aim of the national survey was to measure this temperature. The adopted technique had to satisfy three criteria. First, and most important, it had to be socially acceptable to the respondents. Measuring the temperatures of a random sample of the elderly (quite apart from asking a wide range of questions about income, housing and other factors) was potentially a difficult task. It was important that the techniques used should not make it even more difficult. For example, while the rectal temperature is measured in hospitals, it was unlikely to be acceptable for our purposes. Second, the chosen technique for measuring inner body temperature had to be easy to understand and easy to operate by both interviewer and respondent. Third, the technique had to be relatively inexpensive for a large survey of this kind.

It was fortunate that Dr Fox and his colleagues at the National Institute for Medical Research, Division of Human Physiology, were working on a technique that satisfied the above criteria. In the course of their research a number of possible methods were studied including, for example, the measurement of breath temperature. Some work on the possibility of measuring the temperature of newly passed urine had been done in the past. Following on from this Fox developed the 'uritemp' bottle, which he has described as follows:—

> Essentially it consists of a plastic screw top bottle with a funnel. Urine passes down the funnel over the thermometer bulb and overflows from holes in the upper part of the funnel. Since the thermometer is the usual clinical mercury and glass type it can be read at any time after the urine has been voided[1].

Hand temperature

A special technique was also devised by Fox for the measurement of the temperature of the hand. The purpose was to measure the deep hand temperature and not the skin temperature. As Fox has stated:—

> The reason for this was the realisation that skin temperatures change quite quickly in response to draughts and the environmental conditions, whereas the deep hand temperature is much more consistent as an indicator of the temperature state of the shell of the body[2].

The device consisted of a block of expanded polystyrene with a groove down one side into which a clinical thermometer was positioned and held in place by an elastic band. When correctly positioned the tip of the thermometer protruded from the block touching the palm of the hand. The temperature is recorded after the block has been held for five minutes.

Mouth temperature

Mouth temperatures were measured using a low-reading clinical thermometer. Having checked that the mercury column in the thermometer has been shaken down to the bottom of the scale, the thermometer is placed in the subject's mouth well under the tip of the tongue. It is then left in position with the mouth closed for five minutes. After removal the thermometer is read immediately and the temperature recorded to the nearest 0.01°C.

Environmental temperatures

Living-room and bedroom temperatures were measured, as well as the outdoor temperature. By 'living-room' we meant the room generally lived in by the old person during the day, whatever that room happened to be called. The living-room temperature and the outdoor temperature (i.e. the temperature just outside the house of the respondent) were measured with a whirling hygrometer. In the bedroom, temperatures were measured by means of a maximum-minimum thermometer.

Temperature measurement schedule

Nurses made two visits, one in the late afternoon/early evening and one early the next morning. During the evening visit the measurements of mouth and hand temperatures were taken simultaneously for five minutes. During this time the room temperature was measured using the whirling hygrometer. The subject was asked to use the Uritemp bottle if able to pass a specimen of urine. If not, the Uritemp bottle was left for use as soon as possible (and the subject was asked to note the time of use). A second bottle was left for the following morning (the time again being noted). The maximum-minimum thermometer was placed in a suitable position in the bedroom (or any other room where the person slept). The outdoor temperature was also taken. The next morning the mouth, hand and living-room temperatures were again measured. The morning Uritemp bottle was collected and the maximum-minimum thermometer read and recorded. On leaving the house the outdoor temperature was measured.

The Survey: Methodology

The main objectives of this study were to estimate the size of the 'old and cold' problem – the numbers with low body and room temperatures – and to investigate the socio-economic and environmental characteristics of the 'at risk' group. These objectives largely dictated the study's methodologies. A national, random sample survey of all old people living in private households was essential. However, the nature of the problem – its multidisciplinary aspects – meant that the survey was likely to be more difficult to organize and complete successfully (with an adequate response rate) than most. It involved not only the collection of a variety of information about the circumstances of a sample of the elderly, but also the accurate measurement of body and environmental temperatures. And while temperatures would be measured by equipment that had been designed to be relatively simple and easy to operate, some of it would be strange and new to both survey respondent and fieldworker alike. This put a higher premium than usual on the training and briefing of interviewers. All these considerations made it necessary to give an even greater emphasis to the pilot stage than is normal in survey research.

Pilot Surveys

National pilot survey

A particular task at the pilot stage was to discover whether the chosen techniques could be used in a sample survey of the elderly, while maintaining adequate supervision. Accordingly, the sample was selected in the same way as that later employed in the main survey (described later).

For several reasons the decision was taken to employ nurses as interviewers. Firstly, nurses would be likely to be acquainted with the hypothermia problem and would be skilled at taking, reading and recording body temperatures. Secondly, old people were more likely to cooperate in the research if asked to do so by nurses. Finally, there was every reason to suppose that nurses could be taught how to conduct a social survey. Nurses were recruited locally and briefings carried out. Control and supervision were maintained by the Field Manager and Regional Officers of Opinion Research Centre.

This pilot survey was carried out in two parts. The first, carried out in November, 1970, involved one hundred old people from fifteen randomly selected sampling points in London and the Home Counties. These parts of the country were chosen to ensure maximum possible supervision at this early stage of the project.

During this 'mini-pilot' urine samples were required of men only, whereas, by the time of the main pilot stage, a device had been developed to record the urine temperatures of women also. After this initial series of interviews the questionnaire was slightly modified.

In the main stage of this pilot a national random sample of over three hundred old people were surveyed at different sampling points throughout Great Britain during January, February and March 1971. The pilot confirmed that is was possible to recruit and train nurses to carry out a survey of this type. But the response rate − 62% − was lower than would be needed in the main survey. Nevertheless, the variation between different nurse-interviewers indicated that the low response rate was often due to personality, rather than technical problems. It was felt that the success rate could be improved by increased supervision in the field; by the use of highly experienced interviewers to make the initial appointments; and by embarking on a more ambitious training programme prior to the start of the fieldwork. In the main survey a response rate in the region of 70% would be required, although the results of the pilot suggested that it was unlikely to go very much above this figure. This was due to the reluctance of some old people (who felt that they were perfectly fit!) to participate in this survey; a reluctance by others to give urine samples; and the relative length and nature of the questionnaire (which included questions on income).

Once the old people had agreed to participate, there were no major problems affecting the completion of the questionnaire. Apart from those subjects who found it difficult to pass the necessary amount of urine, only 18 subjects refused to cooperate in the measurement of the urine temperature. One problem concerned the nurses' recording of temperature levels. In spite of a thorough briefing, urging the nurses to make accurate readings of the thermometers, the results of the pilot showed a clear tendency to 'round' to the nearest whole figure. A more detailed briefing and an emphasis on the need to use a magnifying glass when reading thermometers would, it was felt, help to solve this problem.

Portsmouth pilot

Before the national hypothermia survey was fully formulated, a study of body temperatures of the elderly was being planned by Dr Fox and his colleagues from the National Institute for Medical Research in collaboration with Louise Davies of the Geriatric Nutrition Unit at Queen Elizabeth College. It seemed sensible to use this as an opportunity to pilot techniques for the measuring of hand and urine temperatures that were to be used in the main enquiry. As in the other pilot a questionnaire was completed and body and environmental temperatures were taken. Nurses were employed as interviewers. The subjects were chosen from three hundred people over 65 years receiving 'meals on wheels' in Portsmouth in 1971 who had previously taken part in a nutrition survey. One hundred were selected from the nutrition survey to provide a sample stratified by age and sex. The Portsmouth survey took place between 18 January and 10 March 1971 and its results have been published in a separate paper[3].

Lessons from the pilot surveys

Several lessons were learnt from the pilot studies. The most obvious and important was that a 'problem' of low temperatures did exist for the elderly. In both pilot studies a significant proportion of subjects were found to have low body temperatures and, similarly, room temperatures were often found to be low. For example, in the Portsmouth study 22 (15%) of the mouth temperature readings were below 35.5°C. This confirmed the need for a national survey.

The pilot surveys also showed that such a national survey was feasible. Fieldwork could be organized and adequately supervised; and nurses could be recruited and trained. Furthermore, the pilots showed that old people were willing to take part in a survey of this unusual nature despite the demands on their time and the level of cooperation required.

The national pilot had also thoroughly tested a questionnaire which, after amendment, could be confidently used in the national survey. Most importantly, the pilots showed that the techniques used to measure body and environmental temperatures were effective for fieldwork. This was a particularly important finding in relation to the Uritemp bottle for which the pilot studies offered the first major field-trial. In fact the Uritemp bottle was being developed as the pilots were in progress and, in particular, a bottle suitable for females was designed at this stage. The pilots had thus provided an opportunity for research *and development*.

A key lesson of the pilots was the importance of the briefing sessions for the nurse-interviewers. It was necessary to make briefings even more thorough for the major enquiry. Similarly, closer supervision was required.

National Survey

Sample design

The subjects for the national enquiry were selected at random by a systematic probability sample method. A basic sampling point was defined as a parliamentary constituency and the electoral register was used as the basis of the sampling frame. All the constituencies in Great Britain were stratified according to the following criteria:—

a) Registrar-General's Standard Region;
b) the nature of the constituency, i.e. conurbation, borough or county seat;
c) the ratio of Conservative to Labour votes in the 1970 General Election.

A systematic probability sample of 100 constituencies was selected with probability of selection proportionate to size. The proportion of the population aged 65 or over was derived from Registrar-General's and census returns. A sufficient number of names was underlined to yield a total sample of approximately 1,000 persons aged 65 or over. All the names underlined were contacted during October–November and those eligible were told that a nurse would call on them in the New Year. This difficult and expensive way of sampling was used as the best method of obtaining a representative sample throughout Great Britain.

Questionnaire

We needed to enquire into the social and economic circumstances of our elderly respondents and also into their perceptions of thermal conditions. Accordingly a fairly lengthy questionnaire was necessary. However, we were fortunate in being able to draw on the experience and findings of other researchers. In particular we would acknowledge the work of Shanas, Townsend and others in their cross-national survey of the elderly[4]. The questions concerning thermal comfort were based, in part, on the work of Watts[5].

While our national survey was extensive, there were two important areas that we deliberately did not cover: expenditure on heating and nutrition. After careful consideration, both these topics were excluded because of methodological difficulties which could only be avoided by extending our survey (and therefore our questionnaire) to such an extent that its successful completion would be jeopardized. Regarding spending on heating, we concluded that it was not possible to collect reliable information in the course of just two visits to each person. The reasons for this are discussed in Chapter 6 (p.88). Nutritional issues posed even more difficult problems. Clearly the relationship between under-nutrition and low body temperature is an important area for research. However, we were advised by both independent experts and specialists in the Department of Health and Social Security that nutritional aspects could not be tackled in the survey that we were planning. It was certainly not a simple matter of asking a few questions about the number of meals eaten and so on, but rather involved the mounting of a carefully controlled and sophisticated nutritional study. And again this issue could not be tackled in a survey that required just two visits to each person.

Briefing

Nurses were recruited in each locality to carry out the interviews and to take the temperature measurements. They were briefed in groups of up to 20 at a time by staff from Opinion Research Centre and members of the research team (a doctor always being present). The briefings were carried out at seven different centres in England and Scotland during December 1971. Every question in the questionnaire was considered in turn and the use of the hypothermia kit and other techniques were described in detail. The nurse-interviewers were given supervised practice in the techniques. The medical member of the team took great care to stress the need to handle the interviews sensitively, and in the event of an abnormally low body temperature being found, the nurses were instructed to inform the person's general practitioner immediately.

Timing of survey

The survey took place during January, February and March 1972. The fieldwork was spread evenly over the three months to ensure that no particular period of time was over- or under-represented. After an initial visit to ask if the subject was willing to cooperate, morning and evening visits were made as close as possible to set times (8-10 a.m. and 4-6 p.m.).

Two points should be mentioned about the timing of our survey.

Weather conditions

The first concerns the weather conditions during the fieldwork period. Mean environmental temperatures for the survey period were obtained from the Meteorological Office and compared with a 25-year average. This showed that the weather was milder than normal (See table 3.1).

Table 3.1
Average Outdoor Temperatures (°C) during the Survey Period

		January	February	March
England and Wales	) 1972	4.5	5.0	7.0
	) Previous 25 years	4.3	4.5	6.4
Scotland	) 1972	4.1	4.3	5.7
	) Previous 25 years	3.5	3.9	5.4

Source: Meteorological Office.

Miners' strike

During the survey period a miners' strike took place which lasted from 9th January to 28th February 1972. How did this affect our results? Our general impression is that the effect was not considerable. Before the strike was announced we had already included the following question in our survey: 'Do you ever have any trouble getting fuel?' If the answer to this question was 'Yes', details were then sought. After the strike was announced we specially briefed our interviewers to probe for any effects from the strike as part of this question. Our results show that only 63 people (6 per cent) in the sample of over 1,000 reported ever having any trouble getting fuel. Of these, 37 gave the strike as a reason for not getting coal and 5 mentioned electricity power cuts. This evidence strongly suggests that the miners' strike had only a neglible effect on our sample and, in any case, needs to be balanced against the efforts made at this time to get scarce fuel to the elderly and others in need. Also the strike only effected 6 of the 12 weeks of our survey.

Response rate

A total of some 1,342 people aged 65 and over were visited and asked to co-operate in the national survey, of whom 1,020 agreed – a response rate of 76%. Given the nature of the research (involving two visits, a lengthy questionnaire and the measurement of a number of temperatures, including that of urine) and the fact that the nurses were generally inexperienced as interviewers, this was considered to be a very satisfactory response rate.

The national sample

How representative was the sample of the elderly population in general? A comparison of some of the main characteristics of the 1972 survey respondents and data from the 1971 Census is given in the table below. This shows that our sample was reasonably representative in terms of sex, marital status and age distribution.

Table 3.2

Characteristics of the 1972 National Sample and the Population aged 65 and over in 1971 (Percentages)

	1972 Sample	1971 Census*
Sex		
Male	38	38
Female	62	62
Marital Status		
Married	47	49
Single	10	12
Widowed	41	38
Divorced	2	1
Age		
65–69	37	37
70–74	31	27
75–79	17	18
80–84	9	11
85+	6	6

* Source: Office of Population Censuses and Surveys, *Census 1971 Great Britain*. Age, Marital Condition and General Tables, H.M.S.O., 1974 (Based on Table 6).

Processing and analysis of results

Most of the questions used in the survey were pre-coded on the questionnaire but, for some, post-coding was necessary. This was carried out by Opinion Research Centre in consultation with the Centre for Environmental Studies. The checking and analysis of temperature data was carried out at the National Institute for Medical Research under the supervision of Miss Woodward. All temperatures were screened to exclude values that were clearly not reflecting true situations (fevers: if the urine and mouth temperatures were both 38.0°C or more and the hand was not cold all clinical data for the subject were omitted). Notes about the exclusion of temperatures are to be found at the foot of the appropriate tables in Chapter 4. An early computer analysis of data was undertaken at the N.I.M.R. (under Miss Woodward's supervision) and a later analysis was carried out by Opinion Research Centre. Where appropriate, statistical tests of significance were carried out using the chi-square (χ^2) test. Significant differences are shown in the tables as p values. Non-significant differences are denoted by the letters N.S.

Results

Chapter 4
Body and Environmental Temperatures

The first part of this book examined the background to our research and the methods adopted. We can now turn our attention to the results of the national survey. This chapter will present findings about body and room temperatures and in Chapters 5 and 6 the association between temperature levels and various social circumstances of the elderly will be analysed.

Table 4.1 shows the average body and environmental temperatures for the national sample. More information about most of these temperatures will be presented later in this chapter, but two points can be usefully noted at this stage. Firstly, all the body temperatures measured were on average lower for the morning than for the late afternoon/evening visit. This confirms the importance of the circadian rhythm. Secondly, average urine temperatures were higher than average mouth temperatures (and, of course, both were above average hand temperatures). This demonstrates

Table 4.1
Average Body and Environmental Temperatures (± Standard Deviation) in the Morning and Afternoon

	Time	°C	°F
Mouth	a.m.	36.02 ± 0.71	96.84 ± 1.27
	p.m.	36.47 ± 0.52	97.65 ± 0.93
Urine	a.m.	36.28 ± 0.51	97.30 ± 0.92
	p.m.	36.64 ± 0.59	97.95 ± 1.06
Hand	a.m.	31.92 ± 3.03	89.46 ± 5.45
	p.m.	33.65 ± 2.51	92.57 ± 4.52
Living-room	a.m.	15.97 ± 3.38	60.75 ± 6.08
	p.m.	18.16 ± 3.27	64.69 ± 5.88
Outdoor	a.m.	6.99 ± 3.37	44.58 ± 6.07
	p.m.	7.78 ± 3.82	46.00 ± 6.88

the importance of measuring the core temperature. Both of these points can be seen clearly from the summary of the data on body temperatures presented in Figure 4.1.

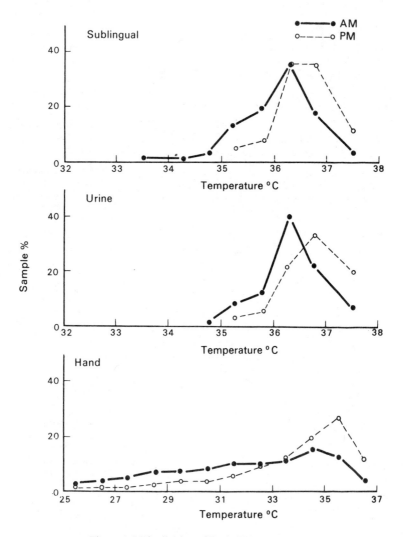

Figure 4.1 Distribution of Body Temperatures

Mouth temperatures

Table 4.2 shows the distribution of mouth temperatures. They were measured sub-lingually, and recorded on the evening and morning visits. According to conventional definitions, large proportions of the sample had 'low' mouth temperatures: almost 20% had temperatures below 35.5°C in the morning and 5% were below 35°C. For the evening, over 5% were below 35.5°C, but fewer than 1% under 35°C.

Viewed on their own, given the emphasis placed on mouth temperatures by some commentators in the past, these findings appear to be very alarming. However, as we argued earlier, the more crucial temperature is that of the deep body (in the case of our survey, the urine temperature) and the mouth temperature results are best evaluated in the context of this. Nevertheless, we can note that a low sub-lingual temperature represents a warning signal and indicates that the core temperature should be measured.

Hand temperatures

Hand temperatures were measured using the method described in Chapter 3. The distribution of these is given in Table 4.3 and it is a very different

Table 4.2

Distribution of Sub-lingual Temperatures: A.M. and P.M.

		A.M.		P.M.	
°F	°C	No.	%	No.	%
Under 87.8	Under 31.0	1	*	–	–
87.8 < 89.6	31.0 < 32.0	1	*	–	–
89.6 < 91.4	32.0 < 33.0	4	*	–	–
91.4 < 93.2	33.0 < 34.0	8	1	2	*
93.2 < 94.1	34.0 < 34.5	12	1	1	*
94.1 < 95.0	34.5 < 35.0	26	3	1	*
95.0 < 95.9	35.0 < 35.5	141	14	48	5
95.9 < 96.8	35.5 < 36.0	193	19	82	8
96.8 < 97.7	36.0 < 36.5	369	36	370	36
97.7 < 98.6	36.5 < 37.0	182	18	367	36
98.6 < 100.4	37.0 < 38.0	39	4	125	12
100.4 and Over	38.0 and Over	2	*	3	*
	Unrecorded or excluded	42	4	21	2
Total		1020	100	1020	100

Effect of hot drinks on mouth temperature: data were excluded if a drink had been taken within half an hour of the temperature being measured and the temperature recorded was more than 1.0°C higher than the urine.

one from that for mouth temperatures. In general, hand temperatures were lower than mouth temperatures. This was to be expected for a surface temperature.

Table 4.3

Distribution of Hand Temperatures: A.M. and P.M.

		A.M.		P.M.	
°F	°C	No.	%	No.	%
Under 77.0	Under 25.0	4	*	2	*
77 < 78.8	25.0 < 26.0	31	3	12	1
78.8 < 80.6	26.0 < 27.0	39	4	11	1
80.6 < 82.4	27.0 < 28.0	52	5	9	1
82.4 < 84.2	28.0 < 29.0	70	7	26	3
84.2 < 86.0	29.0 < 30.0	76	7	37	4
86.0 < 87.8	30.0 < 31.0	77	8	42	4
87.8 < 89.6	31.0 < 32.0	99	10	64	6
89.6 < 91.4	32.0 < 33.0	97	10	91	9
91.4 < 93.2	33.0 < 34.0	114	11	121	12
93.2 < 95.0	34.0 < 35.0	149	15	204	20
95.0 < 96.8	35.0 < 36.0	134	13	270	27
96.8 and Over	36.0 and Over	46	4	118	12
	Unrecorded or excluded	32	3	13	1
Total		1020	100	1020	101

Data were excluded if the hand temperature was more than 0.5°C above both the corresponding mouth and urine temperatures (hand temperatures below 24.0°C had not been recorded by the nurses).

Urine temperatures

In Chapter 1 we discussed the meaning of the term 'hypothermia' and stressed the importance of measuring the inner body or core temperature for its diagnosis. When considering methods in Chapter 3, we briefly described Fox's method of measuring the temperature of urine which we used in the survey. As explained, this method worked well, and approximately 96 per cent of the sample had their urine temperature measured in the morning and approximately 98 per cent the previous evening.

Table 4.4 shows the distribution of urine temperatures. We have already noted that body temperatures are on average higher in the evening than during the morning and this difference is very noticeable when we look at the number of abnormally low urine temperatures. There were 14 old people with temperatures below 35°C in the morning, compared to only 1 the previous evening.

Because of this circadian rhythm, probably exacerbated as we shall see later by the extremely cold night-time conditions experienced by many elderly, we need to focus on those old people with low urine temperatures in the morning. And it is also important to distinguish between those who can be defined as cases of hypothermia and the much larger group who we term as being 'at risk' of developing hypothermia. But, given the distribution of urine temperatures shown in Table 4.4, how many of the

Table 4.4
Distribution of Urine Temperatures*: A.M. and P.M.

		A.M.		P.M.	
°F	°C	No.	%	No.	%
Under 89.6	Under 32.0	1	*	–	–
89.6 < 93.2	32.0 < 34.0	–	–	–	–
93.2 < 94.1	34.0 < 34.5	5	*	–	–
94.1 < 95.0	34.5 < 35.0	8	1	1	*
95.0 < 95.9	35.0 < 35.5	84	8	27	3
95.9 < 96.8	35.5 < 36.0	120	12	65	6
96.8 < 97.7	36.0 < 36.5	404	40	221	22
97.7 < 98.6	36.5 < 37.0	225	22	341	33
98.6 < 100.4	37.0 < 38.0	69	7	199	20
100.4 and Over	38.0 and Over	1	*	2	*
	Unrecorded or excluded	103	10	164	16
Total		1020	100	1020	100

* Data were excluded if the urine volume was less than 50 ml. If the volume was between 50 and 99 ml the data were included if the temperature was (a) greater than 35.5°C or (b) less than 35.0°C and the mouth and hand temperatures were correspondingly low. Data were also excluded if the urine temperature was at least 2.0°C lower than the mouth in the morning or at least 1.0°C lower in the afternoon (a wider limit had to be set for morning data as some collections were made earlier than recommended (8–10 a.m.)).

sample could be said to be suffering from hypothermia in the morning? As can be seen from our preliminary report[1], our definition was a rigorous one. Our starting point can be said to be the 14 persons with temperatures below 35°C. However, this cut-off point is for temperatures measured rectally and Fox et al[2] have shown that the corresponding urine temperature is approximately 34.8°C. Also a number of subjects had mouth temperatures more than 1.0°C above their urine temperatures, and these were excluded. (A low urine temperature in subjects with a falsely high mouth temperature – due, for example, to a recent hot drink – could still have indicated hypothermia, but there was no way of distinguishing this group from those in whom the low urine temperature was the result of a fault in technique.) This left four subjects in our national sample who had urine temperatures of 34.8°C or below (and two with temperatures of 34.8°C to 35.0°C). The hypothermia subjects, so defined, represented 0.58% of the national sample. While this is a very small proportion of the total sample, given the dangers of this condition, it is by no means an insignificant one. It is important to stress the inevitable arbitrary nature of the definition of hypothermia. As we stated in the preliminary report:

> Although the choice of 35.0°C as the lower limit of normality is partly justified by clinical experience, we have shown that individuals can have deep body temperatures fluctuating above and below this arbitrary level, and thus the classification of hypothermia would depend on the time of day that the temperature is taken.

> We therefore believe that it is most unwise to make firm projections of the incidence of hypothermia for the population as a whole. Furthermore, the hypothermia in our . . . subjects is based on a temperature difference of 0.2°C, which clearly has relatively little biological significance[3].

Apart from those with deep body temperature so low that hypothermia can be said to exist (albeit subject to the cautions above), we were anxious to consider those that might be 'at risk' of developing this condition. For this purpose we took 35.5°C (95.9°F) as our cut-off point, and there were 98 persons with morning urine temperatures below this level − 9.6% of the total. In fact this figure is likely to be an underestimate of the numbers 'at risk' at the time of our research because it is a proportion of those surveyed and this includes a number who did not have their urine temperatures measured. In later discussion and tables, this 'at risk' or 'low' urine temperature group (<35.5°C), is compared to a 'normal' group (≥ 36.0°C, excluding fevers). But why do we consider this group to be 'at risk'? In part it is because of the small reserves of body heat possessed by these people. Also (again from our preliminary report):

> The mean urine temperature for the low group was 35.1°C and that for the normal group 36.5°C, so that the core to periphery temperature gradient was 2.9°C in the low group and 4.6°C in the normal group. This indicates a degree of thermo-regulatory inadequacy in the low group compared with the normal group[4].

The 9.6% of the elderly sample who were 'at risk' at the time of the interviews represent over the country as a whole approximately 700,000 people (although this estimate is subject to a margin of error).

Thus the number of old people with unacceptably low deep body temperatures is extremely large. And, as we have noted earlier, our survey was carried out in a winter that was milder than normal. In a severe winter the proportions of the elderly 'at risk' could rise dramatically, as could the numbers suffering from hypothermia.

Room temperatures

How warm or cold were the houses of the old at the time of our survey? Based on the methods described in Chapter 3 we can present findings here on both living-room and bedroom temperatures. In the conclusion to this chapter we will discuss the relationship between body and environmental temperatures.

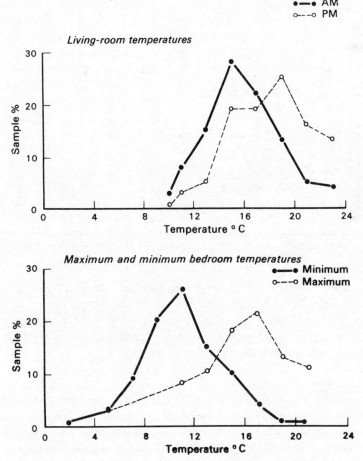

Figure 4.2 Distribution of Living-room and Bedroom Temperatures

Much of the discussion concerning the 'old and cold' problem has focused on the effect of low temperatures on the health of old people. It is important however to discuss the specific problem of hypothermia in a much wider context by looking at room temperatures. Most old people live in dwellings with temperatures below recommended levels and many are in rooms that younger age groups would find intolerably cold, although the young are much more resistant to cold conditions. That cold housing is an important social problem in its own right needs to be emphasized. The distribution of room temperatures found in our survey are summarized in Figure 4.2. In our survey living-room temperatures were measured on both visits: once in the early evening (4–6 p.m.), once the next morning (8–10 a.m.). The distribution of temperatures found in the national sample

Table 4.5
Distribution of A.M. and P.M. Living-room Temperatures

		A.M.		P.M.	
°C	°F	No.	%	No.	%
At or below 10	At or below 50.0	25	3	5	*
10.1 − 12	50.0 − 53.6	82	8	31	3
12.1 − 14	53.6 − 57.2	152	16	52	5
14.1 − 16	57.2 − 60.8	279	28	185	19
16.1 − 18	60.8 − 64.4	217	22	189	19
18.1 − 20	64.4 − 68.0	127	13	253	25
20.1 − 22	68.0 − 71.6	53	5	158	16
22.1 − 24	71.6 − 75.2	44	4	120	13
Total		979	99	993	100

In addition to the above, 41 of the sample in the morning and 27 in the afternoon/evening had temperatures that were unrecorded or excluded.

is shown in Table 4.5. There are several standards with which to compare these results. The highest is one that used to be recommended by the Department of Health and Social Security in its leaflet 'Keeping Warm in Winter' (1972) which states: 'To keep old people warm in winter the living-room temperature should be about 70°F when the temperature outside is 30°F. Bathrooms and bedrooms should be kept at the same temperature if possible, but in any event should be kept warm.'*

Another standard is found in the Parker Morris Report of 1961 which laid down a minimum level of 18.3°C (65.0°F). Considering morning temperatures first we can see from the table that 90% had living-room temperatures at or below 68°F − i.e. 2°F below the DHSS recommended level;

*The withdrawal of this recommendation is discussed in Chapter 9, pp. 140–41.

76% had temperatures at or below 64.4°F – i.e. 0.6°F below the Parker Morris recommendation. Most temperatures were therefore way below these recommended levels. In fact 54% of room temperatures were at or below 16.0°C (60.8°F), the minimum temperature specified in the Offices, Shops and Railway Premises Act of 1963. In other words most of the elderly experienced morning temperatures which Parliament had felt to be too low for (generally younger) office workers and other employees.

The distribution of early evening room temperatures differs from the morning ones. Living-room temperatures were naturally higher – the average morning temperature was 15.97°C (60.7°F) compared to the average evening temperature of 18.16°C (64.67°F). However, what is interesting here is the continuance of generally low temperature levels. The vast majority of old persons had living-room temperatures below the DHSS recommended level – 71% were at or below 68°F. A large proportion were below the Parker Morris recommended level – 46% were at or below 64.4°F. Twenty-seven per cent were at or below the level laid down by the 1963 Act which employers can be prosecuted for not maintaining.

The results outlined above show that the majority of old people in Britain are living in rooms with lower temperatures than those recommended. Substantial proportions have living-room temperatures that are cruelly low.

We were also interested in bedroom temperatures. This is likely to be a particularly important factor given the importance of the early morning urine temperatures. Our nurse-interviewers placed a maximum-minimum thermometer in the bedroom (or any other room where the person slept) during the evening visit and the two temperature measurements were recorded the next day during the early morning visit.

As with living-rooms, the temperatures of bedrooms were generally low. However, as might be expected, they were much lower than for living-rooms. The results are given in Table 4.6. Taking the distribution of minimum temperatures, it can be seen that 4% of the sample had bedroom temperatures below 6°C (42.8°F); 33% were below 10°C (50°F) and 84% were below 16°C (60.8°F). Only 16 people had minimum temperatures at or above 20°C (68°F). As previously mentioned, the DHSS had recommended bedroom temperatures for the elderly of 70°F. The distribution of maximum bedroom temperatures, although of course higher, confirms the picture of generally cold conditions (39% being below 16°C).

In later analysis we will concentrate on two particular room temperatures: morning living-room and minimum bedroom. Some selection of data was necessary, but we focus on these two for particular reasons. The effect of the circadian rhythm is that body temperatures are lower at night and in the morning and rise during the day. This suggested that we should

focus our enquiries on the period when body temperatures are lowest. Our
tables on room temperatures also include an analysis of those who experienced the coldest living-room temperatures (i.e. below 14°C (57.2°F)) in

Table 4.6

Distribution of Bedroom Temperatures

		Minimum		Maximum	
°F	°C	Temperatures		Temperatures	
Up to 39.0	Up to 3.9°	12	1%		
39.1 − 42.6	4 − 5.9°	28	3%	31	3%
42.7 − 46.2	6 − 7.9°	96	9%		
46.3 − 49.8	8 − 9.9°	203	20%		
49.9 − 53.4	10 − 11.9°	269	26%	84	8%
53.5 − 57.0	12 − 13.9°	152	15%	100	10%
57.1 − 60.6	14 − 15.9°	99	10%	180	18%
60.7 − 64.2	16 − 17.9°	43	4%	215	21%
64.3 − 67.8	18 − 19.9°	14	1%	135	13%
67.9 − 71.4	20 − 21.9°	11	1%	108	11%
71.5 and above	22°C and above	5	*%	83	8%
	Unrecorded or excluded	88	9%	84	8%
Total		1020	100%	1020	100%

both the morning and the late afternoon/evening. There were 56 old
people in this group − some 5% of the sample. This group is of particular
interest, because the two sets of living-room temperature data suggest that
their homes remain cold throughout the day.

Cold conditions and body temperatures

What do our survey findings tell us about the relationship between body
and room temperatures? At the outset of our research we had two
hypotheses − indeed really basic assumptions − in mind about temperatures. First it was felt that the different body temperatures measured
would correlate with one another. Second, we expected to find an association between body and room temperatures: in particular we had assumed
that those with the lowest deep body temperatures would be living in the
coldest conditions. This last point seemed almost self-evident and it lies in
the background of much of the public discussion about the old and cold.

Do our survey findings − summarized in Table 4.7 − bear out these
assumptions? The results do confirm that there is a general relationship

between body temperatures (the exception being the non-significant relationship between urine and hand temperature in the morning). The data on hand temperatures are also interesting. As we stated in the preliminary report: 'The significant correlations found between the hand and all the

Table 4.7

Correlation Between Temperatures

	Time of Day	All Respondents
Mouth/Urine	a.m.	**
	p.m.	**
Mouth/Hand	a.m.	**
	p.m.	**
Urine/Hand	a.m.	N.S.
	p.m.	**
Mouth/Living-room	a.m.	**
	p.m.	**
Urine/Living-room	a.m.	N.S.
	p.m.	N.S.
Hand/Living-room	a.m.	**
	p.m.	**
Mouth/Outdoor	a.m.	**
	p.m.	N.S.
Urine/Outdoor	a.m.	N.S.
	p.m.	N.S.
Hand/Outdoor	a.m.	**
	p.m.	N.S.
Living-room/Outdoor	a.m.	**
	p.m.	**

N.S. = Not significant
** = $P < 0.01$
Source: This table is based on Table V, R. H. Fox *et al,* 'Body Temperatures in the Elderly: A National Study of Physiological, Social, and Environmental Conditions.' *British Medical Journal,* 27 January 1973.

other temperatures reflect the important role of the peripheral parts of the body in thermoregulatory control[5].' But how do cold conditions affect body temperatures? Here there is a surprise. Although there is the expected significant association between living-room temperatures and mouth and hand temperatures, there is *no* significant association between room temperatures and urine temperatures. As we stated in our preliminary report: 'This indicates that for the group as a whole the thermoregulatory mechanisms were maintaining deep body temperature homeostasis . . .[6].' In layman's terms our results confirm that cold conditions do adversely affect the elderly and consequently temperatures on the body's surface do drop, but, in general, natural defences maintain adequate warmth within the body. This lack of association between room temperatures and urine temperatures is an extremely interesting finding and has important implications for the analysis of other data from the national survey. It is therefore worth analysing in more detail, and Table 4.8 presents data on the distribution of living-room and minimum bedroom temperatures for both 'normal' and 'low' urine temperature groups.

This confirms the lack of any significant association. Thus, for example, 68% of those with morning living-room temperatures at or below 13°C had normal urine temperatures compared to 69% of those in the 18°C and above living-room temperature group. What are the implications of this unexpected result for our study? It certainly does not mean that cold conditions do not cause low deep body temperatures. As we have shown most of the elderly experience morning living-room and minimum bedroom temperatures which are below recommended standards. And, as can be seen from Table 4.8, most of the low urine temperature group lived in cold conditions. In fact of the 98 people in this group only 4 had minimum bedroom temperatures above 16°C (60.8°F) while temperatures at or below 12°C (53.6°F) were experienced by 59 old people. So although living in very cold conditions does not necessarily lead to low deep body temperatures, the group 'at risk' do, in general, live in cold conditions.

Nevertheless, our results show a minority of cases where it appears that low deep body temperatures are probably not caused by cold conditions — for example the 4 'at risk' elderly people with minimum bedroom temperatures of 16°C or above (of which 2 were between 20 and 21°C). It is reasonable to look for a non-environmental or endogenous cause of low deep body temperature in such cases. Examples of such causes might be an illness or the use of certain drugs which affect the thermoregulatory system.* Our national survey was not intended to investigate the causes of endogenous hypothermia. We were concerned rather with what it can be reasonably argued is the common cause of hypothermia or low body temperatures — cold conditions. Our data on room temperatures show that this is the common factor and the significant relationship between room temperatures and surface body temperatures confirms this. But we have shown that most of the old living in cold conditions are able to maintain deep body temperature homeostasis, so why do a minority fail to do so? Is it possible to distinguish any social factors that are associated with the 'at risk' elderly?

*See Chapter 1 for a brief discussion of endogenous cases of hypothermia. Their existence in this survey will however produce 'errors' in any statistical analysis which should be borne in mind.

Table 4.8   Morning Urine Temperatures by Living-room and Minimum Bedroom Temperatures

| | Total | A.M. Living-room Temperature | | | | Cold A.M. and P.M. | Minimum Bedroom Temperature | | | | |
		0–13	14–15	16–17	18+		<8	8<10	10<12	12<16	16+
Total	1,020	242	274	228	237	56	136	203	269	251	73
A.M. Urine Temperature											
Low	98 10%	29 12%	31 11%	17 7%	18 8%	5 9%	13 10%	24 12%	22 8%	25 10%	4 5%
Normal	699 69%	164 68%	194 71%	164 72%	163 69%	40 71%	95 70%	146 72%	188 70%	175 70%	50 68%
			N.S.						N.S.		

In this and subsequent tables, the column headed 'Cold A.M. and P.M.' consists of the 56 people in the sample who had the coldest living rooms (below 14°C/57.2°F) in both the morning and afternoon/evening.
'Total' in this and subsequent tables refers to the sample (1020 respondents). In the case of room temperatures, unrecorded or excluded measurements are not shown. For urine temperatures only the 'low' (<35.5°C) and 'normal' (≥36.0°C) groups are included.

Results

Chapter 5 'At Risk'

In the last chapter it was shown that, according to our definition, one-tenth of our elderly sample were 'at risk' of their inner body temperature falling to a level that, it is commonly accepted, constitutes hypothermia. Our evidence also demonstrates that very large proportions of the elderly live in cold conditions. However, our results do not show any association between low inner body temperatures and low room temperatures (although the latter are associated with mouth and hand temperatures). In other words it is *not* the case that those 'at risk' of hypothermia are so because they inhabit colder homes than others. As we argued in the last chapter this was a surprising finding and has important implications for the analysis of other results.

At the outset of this project our general hypothesis about the 'hypothermia' problem was that in a number – and probably the majority – of cases there would be an exogenous cause. In general, we assumed, those elderly people living in the coldest rooms would be significantly more likely to have low inner body temperatures. The reason for cold conditions might be due to one or a combination of factors such as bad housing, poverty, social isolation, physical immobility and so on.

We have seen that our results do not support the initial part of this explanation concerning inner body and room temperatures. What are the implications of this? In practice we need to investigate two separate questions. First, why do a minority (i.e. those 'at risk') *fail* to maintain deep body temperature homeostasis? Second, what are the socio-economic factors that are associated with low room temperatures? These two questions are, at least to a large extent, separate because it is important to view the existence of cold – often severely cold – living conditions as a social problem in its own right. In certain cases such conditions may jeopardize the health of the individual – and in extreme cases cause death – but we should not only become concerned at this stage.

Not enough attention has been focused on the sheer human misery caused by cold living conditions. The aspect of our investigation relating to this question is pursued in the next chapter. But why do a minority of the elderly have low body temperatures? Are their social circumstances different in important respects from those with normal body temperatures? Conversely are there certain factors that help prevent hypothermia? And do those 'at risk' feel cold or desire warmer conditions? These questions are discussed in this chapter. (The consideration of room temperature levels will be included only where their association with urine temperatures seems possible.)

How do we explain low urine temperatures?

Given that low living-room temperatures do not *necessarily* cause a fall in urine temperature, several possibilities can be pursued. Are the 'at risk' distinguishable in some significant respect from those with normal body temperatures? Or is a physiological factor, rather than a social one, important? Or perhaps there are social factors that have an 'immediate' effect on body temperature, rather than just via environmental temperature.

Having found no significant association between low deep body temperatures and the coldest conditions, it follows that one would *not* now expect significant relationships between the 'at risk' group and certain social or economic factors. For example, if the 'at risk' did live in the coldest dwellings, it might be reasonable to expect that those in the worst housing are more likely to be 'at risk' because inadequate housing might be the coldest. At the very least, given our initial view, it would have been a reasonable hypothesis. But on the basis of our evidence, we would now not expect to find such associations. And this is generally the case as a 'check-list' of findings presented in Table A.1* shows.

There is no significant association between housing tenure, house-type, use of basic amenities or possession of central heating and low urine temperatures in the morning. Similarly, whether or not an old person is living alone or physically immobile has no statistically significant effect on deep body temperature. However, certain factors are significantly associated with those 'at risk'. These are the sex of the individual, age and the receipt of supplementary benefits, and the findings here are presented in Figure 5.1. The first of these three can probably be simply accounted for. There is no reason to expect that sex, per se, is important. Rather the statistical significance of sex is almost certainly related to the findings about age. The life expectancy of females is higher than for males and consequently a higher proportion of the very aged are female.

Regarding age, Figure 5.1 shows the association between age groups and urine temperature levels. Whereas only 28% of those 'at risk' were

*Tables A.1 to A.12 can be found in the Appendix.

aged 65−69, as many as 40% of the 'normal' group were in this age group. At the other extreme 19% of the 'at risk' were aged 80 or over compared to 13% of those with 'normal' temperatures. These differences are statistically significant and consequently it is important to pursue the importance of the age factor. However, at the outset one must warn against exaggerating the significance of age. Our results do not support any simple policy approaches, such as a greater concentration of resources on the over-80s. For while increasing age does appear to increase the chances of being 'at risk' from cold conditions, substantial numbers of those with 'low' body temperatures are relatively young pensioners.

Why is it that, while most of the elderly living in cold conditions − and indeed most of those with low mouth and hand temperatures − are able to maintain a 'normal' urine temperature, a failure to do so increases with age? One obvious explanation − room temperature − can be quickly ruled out. As Table A.10 shows, the very aged were no more likely to be living in the coldest conditions than other, younger, pensioners. Nor, incidentally, were the very aged less likely to have central heating. In fact 23% of those aged 65−69 had central heating compared to 24%: 70−74; 22%: 75−79; 22%: 80−84; and 26% for those aged 85 and over.

There are physiological and medical reasons for the relationship between age and low deep body temperature, but other social factors appear to play a part.

How do we account for the association between low urine temperatures and the receipt of supplementary benefits? As can be seen from Figure 5.1, 50% of the 'at risk' were receiving supplementary benefit compared to only 33% of the normal temperature group. This finding suggests poverty as an explanation but we were rightly cautious about this. Our results in fact show *no* clear association between poverty and room temperatures. Table A.2 gives the distribution of room temperatures by receipt of supplementary pension. This shows *no* association between the receipt of supplementary pension and room temperatures. This seems to rule out a simple explanation that poor people cannot afford warm homes and therefore their body temperatures are more likely to be low. This is confirmed by Table A.3 which shows no clear association between either body or room temperatures and income. For example, for single persons, 38% of those with 'low' urine temperatures had weekly incomes of up to £7.50 compared to 33% of those in the 'normal' temperature group. The income differences between the two groups are not statistically significant. A similar picture emerges for married couples. (The relationship between poverty and cold conditions is discussed in Chapter 6).

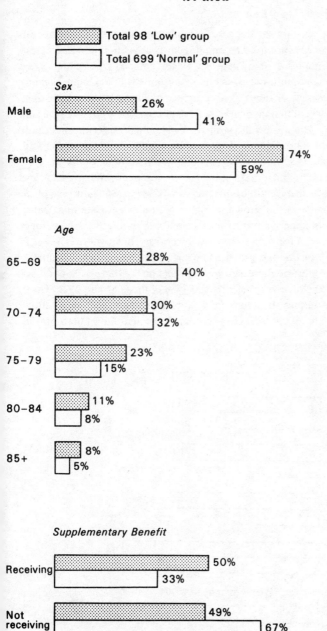

Figure 5.1 Percentages of 'Low' and 'Normal' Urine Temperature Groups (A.M.)
by Sex, Age and Supplementary Benefit.

Age and Supplementary Benefits

So how do we account for the association between supplementary pensions and the 'at risk' group? Age would seem an obvious explanation. It is known (see Chapter 2) that, generally, supplementary pensioners are older on average than other pensioners and our own data support this. Thirty-one per cent of those aged 65–69 in our sample were receiving supplementary benefits, compared to 33% of those aged 70–74; 34% for those aged 75–79; 45% for those aged 80–84; and 35% for those 85 and over (or 42% for 80 and over). These figures suggest that in the analysis of body temperatures supplementary benefits might be of no importance in their own right, but merely reflect the greater age of beneficiaries. Is this so? It is useful to analyse urine temperatures by both age and the receipt of benefits. This analysis is shown in Figure 5.2 (which is based on Table A.4). This lends some support to the 'age factor' hypothesis, but age does not totally account for the observed differences. Thus, whereas 41% of those 'at risk' in the age group 65–69 were receiving supplementary benefits the proportion increased with age to a point where 64% of those aged 80–84 were receiving benefits and 75% of those 85 and over. Thus age *is* an important explanation of the supplementary benefit association with low urine temperatures. However, the table also shows that, *within*

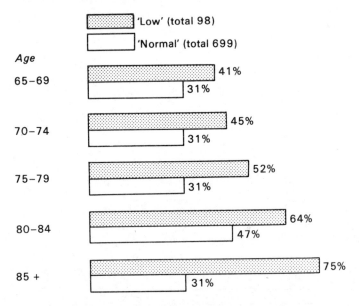

Figure 5.2 Percentages of 'Low' and 'Normal' Urine Temperature Groups (A.M.) receiving Supplementary Benefit by Age.

age groups − and for all age groups − those 'at risk' are more likely to be receiving benefits than those with 'normal' temperatures.

To explore this question further it is useful to present the data in a different way. Table 5.1 shows the proportion who are in the low and normal temperature categories, within age groups, according to whether or not benefit is being received. This shows that, among non-recipients of supplementary benefit, the very aged are *not* more likely to be in the lower temperature group, i.e. 'at risk', than younger pensioners. However, among supplementary benefit recipients, there is a pattern in this direction. Thus, whereas 10 per cent of supplementary benefit recipients aged 65−69 were at risk, the proportion for those aged 85 and over is 26 per cent. On the basis of this evidence then the very old on supplementary benefit are some four times as likely to be at risk of developing hypothermia as, say, elderly people not on supplementary benefit.

A major implication of our result is that, far from the receipt of supplementary benefit being merely an indicator of age, the importance of the age factor is largely explained by the fact that it is the very aged supplementary benefit recipients who are most at risk. Why is this?

Table 5.1

'Low' and 'Normal' Groups by Age and Receipt of Supplementary Benefit

(a) Receiving S.B.

Age	Total	Low No.	%	Normal No.	%	
65 − 69	115	11	10	88	77	
70 − 74	102	13	13	70	69	
75 − 79	61	12	20	34	56	0.05>p>0.02
80 − 84	41	7	17	26	63	
85+	23	6	26	10	43	
Totals	342	49	14	228	67	

(b) Not Receiving S.B.

Age	Total	Low No.	%	Normal No.	%	
65 − 69	257	16	6	191	74	
70 − 74	210	16	8	153	73	
75 − 79	114	11	10	72	63	N.S.
80 − 84	48	3	6	29	60	
85+	40	2	5	20	50	
Totals	669	48	7	465	70	

The answer is not clear, but probably is due to the greater relative deprivation of this group. To consider this it is useful to look at the particular characteristics of supplementary beneficiaries in our sample compared to those of other elderly people. From Table 5.2 it can be seen that there are a number of statistically significant differences between receivers and non-receivers of benefit. Higher proportions of those on benefit are women and beneficiaries are older and more likely to be widowed than others. About half of them live alone compared to only a quarter of other pensioners. Judged by amenities, their housing is no worse than that of others. Seventeen per cent of benefit recipients have central heating (as against 26% of others) while only 30% have electric blankets (compared to 41% of others). The data on observed body weight show no major differences although our interviewers estimated that fewer of the supplementary benefit recipients were of 'normal' weight. One-fifth of beneficiaries receive social welfare callers compared to approximately one-tenth of other pensioners. The picture that emerges from the table confirms the view that benefit recipients are generally deprived compared to other elderly people. And while, as we have shown, poverty itself does not simply relate to low body temperatures, it clearly will be important in some cases and this will be reflected in our data. Whatever the explanation, the results indicate the importance of the system of supplementary benefits and underline the responsibilities that the Supplementary Benefits Commission has in this field (discussed in Chapter 7).

The fact that it is the very aged supplementary beneficiaries who are most at risk is probably due to two groups of factors. Firstly the very aged are in general more deprived than younger pensioners in terms of a number of socio-economic factors (see Chapter 2). Consequently very aged benefit recipients are likely to include some of the most deprived old people in Britain. The second group include physiological or medical factors. In general the human thermoregulatory system becomes less efficient with age and consequently the very aged will sometimes find it more difficult (than younger people) to maintain a normal deep body temperature. The evidence presented in Table 5.1, however suggests that while most of the very aged do maintain a normal temperature, this is less easy in adverse social circumstances. Our evidence would therefore suggest that a combination of a declining physiology (perhaps exacerbated by increasing illness and the effect of drugs) and the most deprived socio-economic conditions will greatly increase the risk of an old person becoming hypothermic.

'Immediate' influences on body temperature

One of the implications of the lack of association between living-room and

Table 5.2

Selected Characteristics of National Sample
by Receipt of Supplementary Benefits

	Total ⌀		Receiving Supplementary Benefits		Not Receiving Supplementary Benefits		
	No.	%	No.	%	No.	%	
Total	1,020	100	342	34	669	66	
Sex							
Male		38		29		43	p<0.001
Female		62		71		57	
Marital Status							
Married		47		32		55	
Single		10		10		10	p<0.001
Widowed		41		57		33	
Divorced/Separated		2		2		1	
Age							
65 – 74		67		63		70	0.05>p>0.02
75+		33		37		30	
Household Composition							
Living alone		34		51		25	p<0.001
Living with other(s)		66		49		75	
Housing							
Exclusive use of all amenities		70		70		70	N.S.
Central Heating							
With		23		17		26	p<0.001
Without		77		83		74	
Electric Blanket							
With		37		30		41	p<0.001
Without		63		70		59	
Weight							
'Very obese'/ 'Obese'		3		5		3	
'Somewhat overweight'		23		25		22	
'Normal'		55		51		58	0.02>p>0.01
'Somewhat underweight'		14		14		14	
'Emaciated'/'Very emaciated'		2		4		1	
*Social Welfare Callers**							
One or more		15		20		11	p<0.001
None		85		80		89	

⌀ In addition to those receiving or not receiving supplementary benefit, there were 9 in the sample who did not respond to this question.

* i.e. domestic/home help; welfare officer; health visitor; meals-on-wheels.

urine temperatures is that, whereas we had originally sought associations between low urine temperatures and socio-economic factors (such as bad housing and poverty) we would now not expect such associations. Where

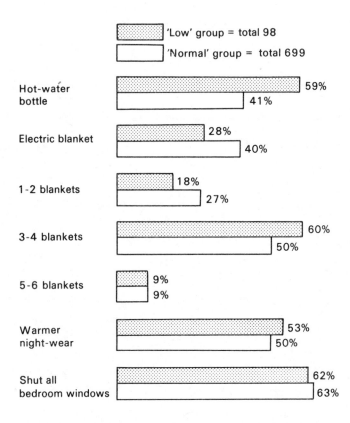

In addition 8% used an eiderdown/bedspread/quilt and 1% used a bedheater/warming pan (all these being in the normal group).
16 respondents mentioned 'other' methods and 3 reported using none of the above.

Figure 5.3 Percentages of 'Low' and 'Normal' Urine Temperature Groups (A.M.) by Methods of Keeping Warm at Night.

associations are found they are probably due to either (a) an association (at least in part) between the factor and 'age', or (b) the fact that there is an *immediate* association with low urine temperatures (and not simply an effect through room temperatures).

As mentioned earlier the receipt of supplementary pensions is in part an example of the type of factor associated with age. Our results also provide examples of factors that might reasonably be expected to have an immediate association with low urine temperatures. It would seem, for example, that night-time 'safeguards' against the cold are associated with morning urine temperatures. Figure 5.3 shows the ways in which the elderly attempt to keep warm at night. Not surprisingly some old people use more than one 'method' to keep warm and, for this reason, an analysis by body temperatures has to be interpreted cautiously: the temperature distribution of any one category (e.g. those wearing warmer nightwear) will be influenced by other measures taken. Nevertheless, some important points emerge from this figure. In particular it appears to be the case that those with electric blankets are more likely to have 'normal' urine temperatures than those with hot-water bottles (who are over-represented in the 'low' group).

A comparison of those using electric blankets and the rest of the sample shows a statistically significant difference between urine temperature distribution of the two groups ($0.05 > p > 0.02$). Only 28% of the 'low' group had electric blankets compared to 40% of the 'normal' group. Thus, although it is not a sure protection against a low body temperature, our evidence strongly suggests that the use of electric blankets is relatively effective in helping the elderly to maintain normal temperatures and preventing hypothermia. But there is a need for caution before accepting this conclusion. Might it not be that the use of electric blankets is strongly associated with age and that our results purely reflect this?

An analysis of the use of electric blankets by age confirms that younger pensioners are more likely to use them than the very aged. In fact 42% of those aged 65–69 used them, compared to 39%: 70–74; 31%: 75–79; 29%: 80–84; and 26%: 85 and over. So does this indicate that electric blankets are not important in their own right?

The analysis in Table 5.3 divides the sample into two groups, those under 75 and those aged 75 and over and it suggests that the use of these blankets has an effect on urine temperatures that is not accounted for by age. Those with low body temperatures were less likely to have electric blankets in both age groups. The difference is most pronounced for the older groups. Here only 14% of those 'at risk' had these blankets, compared to 33% of the 'normal' group.

Another explanation for the apparent importance of electric blankets might simply be that those possessing them were sleeping in warmer bedrooms than others. But our results reported in Table A.5 provide no support for this suggestion. For example, 38% of those with minimum bedroom temperatures below 8°C had electric blankets, and the proportion was the same for those with temperatures of 16°C or above.

Another reason for the observed association between electric blankets and body temperature, might be that such blankets are simply an indicator of greater affluence, but this would seem to be ruled out by our finding that levels of income are not associated with urine temperatures.

The evidence of this survey would therefore seem to indicate a clear relationship between using electric blankets and having a normal urine temperature. It is, of course, important not to overstate this for a proportion of those using electric blankets *were* 'at risk' — their use is no sure protection. They are certainly no substitute for warm bedrooms. However, they do appear to contribute to the effective prevention of hypothermia and the policy implications of this are discussed in our concluding chapter. Nevertheless we can note here that persuading the very aged to use electric blankets would be no easy matter, quite apart from problems of cost and safety.

Table 5.3
Use of Electric Blankets by Age and Urine Temperatures

		Low (98)		Normal (699)	
		%	No.	%	No.
Electric Blankets:					
Yes	65–74	37.5	21	42.3	213
No		62.5	35	57.7	291
			56		504
Yes	75 and over	14.3	6	33.3	65
No		85.7	36	66.6	130
			42		195

Assessment of weight

Another important finding from the survey concerns body weight. We asked the nurse/interviewers to assess the weight of the subject in relation to height. Seven categories ranging from 'very obese' to 'very emaciated' were listed on the questionnaire. A cautionary note is needed here. To categorize a sample of subjects on the basis of interviewers' judgments is bound to be fairly crude and open to error. On the other hand a careful briefing on this aspect of the study was given and in this way it is hoped that variation between interviewers was minimized.

With these important cautions in mind, it is the case that the results are of considerable interest when analysed by temperature levels. As can be seen from Table A.6, 26% of the sample were judged to be 'very obese', 'obese' or 'somewhat overweight', 55%, 'normal', 14% 'somewhat underweight', and 2% 'emaciated' or 'very emaciated'. There were very similar proportions of the 'overweight' in both the normal and low temperature groups. However, as Figure 5.4 shows, there are differences, which are statistically significant, between the group with normal weight and those who were 'somewhat underweight' and those who were 'emaciated' or 'very emaciated'. Thus 6% of the low urine temperature group were 'emaciated' or 'very emaciated' compared to only 1% of the normal temperature group. And while 59% of the normal temperature group were judged to be of normal weight, the figure for the 'at risk' group was only 47%. It is also worth noting that of the nineteen subjects judged to be 'emaciated' or 'very emaciated' six had low urine temperatures in the morning. The numbers here however, are too small to be very confident about the importance of this specific finding.

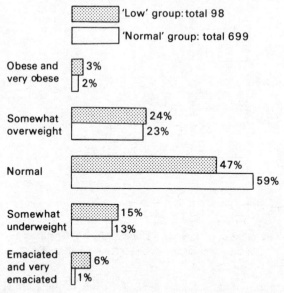

Figure 5.4 Percentages of 'Low' and 'Normal' Urine Temperature Groups (A.M.) by Assessment of Weight.

Why are the emaciated more likely to have low urine temperatures? One possible explanation might be that they are living in colder rooms, but this is not the case as Table A.6 shows. And again we need to investigate the relationship between body weight and age. Do the findings about weight merely reflect our findings about age?

Figure 5.5 analyses the assessment of weight by urine temperatures and by two age groups – those under 75 and those aged 75 and over. This shows that, as expected, the older group did contain a higher proportion of underweight persons. However, it is again the case that age does not account for all the associations. For within both age groups it was more likely for a low temperature group to contain more of those underweight and fewer of those assessed as being of normal weight. For example, in the

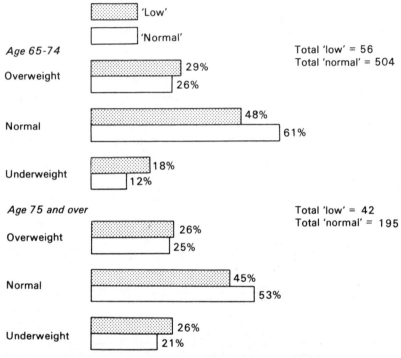

Figure 5.5 Percentages of 'Low' and 'Normal' Urine Temperature Groups (A.M.) for the under and over 75s by Assessment of Weight.

younger pensioner group, only 48% of the low temperature group were assessed as having normal body weight, compared to 61% of those in the normal temperature group. The respective figures for the older age group are 45% and 53%. The data therefore suggest the importance of body weight as an independent influence on body temperature. May this, in part, explain the importance of the age factor in temperature regulation? Michael Green has explained the effect of body weight:—

The temperature of the body core is the critical factor. In smaller and thinner people, and babies, the body core is a relatively larger part of the person, and the surface area is also proportionally larger. In such individuals deep body cooling may occur more quickly and more profoundly in adverse environmental conditions or illness[1].

Although we were not able to study nutrition in this study (for the reasons mentioned in Chapter 3) the findings about body weight indicate its importance in any explanation of hypothermia.

Feelings, Comfort and Preferences

Earlier on in this chapter we argued that where associations were found between certain social factors and urine temperatures this would be due to either a relationship between the factor and age or the fact that there could be an *immediate* association with low urine temperatures. In fact there is a third group of factors that might reasonably be expected to be related to urine temperatures. These factors are old people's feelings and preferences about the cold and warmth.

An important part of our survey was concerned with these matters. We asked questions about 'feeling cold indoors', hand comfort, general body comfort and preferences for warmth. The results of these questions will be analysed by both urine and environmental temperature. Such an analysis will help to throw light on one of the more interesting hypotheses about hypothermia: that the potential victims of this condition sometimes are seemingly unaware of the cold conditions in which they live (or the coldness of their bodies) and will not therefore seek help. The British Medical Association special committee on hypothermia reported that 'patients do not necessarily complain of cold'[2]. Is this view supported by our findings or is it the case that those 'at risk' and those living in the coldest conditions do in fact feel cold more often, feel less comfortable and would prefer more warmth?

Feeling cold indoors

We asked the elderly in our sample, 'Would you say you ever feel cold indoors?' The answers to this question, analysed by temperature levels, are given in Table 5.4. 10% of the sample stated that they felt cold 'very often', while the same proportion felt cold 'fairly often'. At the other extreme 28% 'never' felt cold. An analysis by urine temperatures shows that in general our 'at risk' group *were* more likely to feel cold 'very often' (22%) than the 'normal' group (9%).

Table 5.4

Feeling Cold Indoors by Room and Urine Temperatures

	Total	Minimum Bedroom Temperature					Morning Living-room Temperature				Cold A.M. and P.M.	Urine Temperature A.M.	
		<8	8<10	10<12	12<16	16+	0–13	14–15	16–17	18+		Under 35.5	36.0+
Total:	1,020	136	203	269	251	73	242	274	228	237	56	98	699
Feeling cold indoors?													
1. Very often	10%	12%	13%	9%	7%	8%	16%	9%	9%	8%	27%	22%	9%
2. Fairly often	10%	13%	12%	10%	7%	10%	11%	13%	9%	6%	11%	8%	9%
3. Sometimes	32%	32%	31%	32%	36%	30%	35%	28%	35%	28%	41%	33%	32%
4. Rarely	20%	24%	16%	22%	22%	14%	19%	24%	17%	19%	7%	13%	19%
5. Never	28%	19%	28%	28%	29%	38%	20%	25%	31%	38%	14%	23%	30%
				N.S.					p<0.001			0.005>p >0.001	

A similar picture emerges if one looks at morning living-room temperatures. Thus whereas 27% of those with temperatures below 14°C felt cold 'very often' or 'fairly often', only 14% of those with temperatures of 18°C or above responded in these ways. At the other extreme 20% of those with living-room temperatures below 14°C 'never' felt cold indoors compared to 38% of those with temperatures of 18°C or above. The pattern is more pronounced for the group with the lowest living-room temperatures in both the morning and the evening. Twenty-seven per cent felt cold 'very often' and a further 11% 'fairly often'. There is not such a clear pattern for minimum bedroom temperatures and the differences here are not statistically significant. This is rather surprising, but it is necessary to note the importance of, to take the main example, electric blankets on the warmth of the body at night.

These are the general findings, but the table also clearly shows that large proportions of those in our 'at risk' group and of those living in cold living-rooms reported that they felt cold rarely or never. Thus as many as 23% of the 'at risk' group reported that they 'never' felt cold indoors while a further 13% claimed to feel cold 'rarely'. Similarly, an analysis by living-room temperatures shows that, for the morning, 20% of those with temperatures below 14°C reported 'never' feeling cold indoors. And as many as 43% of those with the coldest bedrooms said that they were 'rarely' or 'never' cold indoors. The implications of these findings are discussed later.

Hand comfort

We asked two questions about the comfort of the hands and the results are given in Table 5.5. The first was simply:'Do your hands ever feel numb or cold indoors?' As can be seen, 39% of the sample replied 'yes' to this question, 60% 'no'. Analysed by urine temperatures it can be seen that there is a significant association between such temperatures and the response to this question. Almost half (49%) of the 'at risk' group did (ever) feel numb or cold indoors, compared to 37% of the 'normal' group. Similarly there is a clear trend for living-room temperatures and it is noticeable that 61% of those with very cold (below 14°C) living-rooms in both the morning and evening reported that their hands felt cold indoors. However there is no very clear picture for bedroom temperatures.

The second question concerning the hands was more detailed and involved the respondents reporting their hand comfort on a scale that ranged from 'much too warm' to 'much too cool'. In fact no one said that their hands were 'much too warm' and only three persons said that they were 'too warm'. Only the main categories are therefore shown in Table

Table 5.5

Hands 'Numb or Cold' and Hand Comfort by Room and Urine Temperatures

	Total	Minimum Bedroom Temperature					Morning Living-room Temperature				Cold A.M. and P.M.	Urine Temperature A.M.	
		<8	8<10	10<12	12<16	16+	0-13	14-15	16-17	18+		Under 35.5	36.0+
Total:	1,020	136	203	269	251	73	242	274	228	237	56	98	699
Hands Numb or Cold?													
Yes	39%	43%	43%	36%	39%	36%	46%	39%	40%	32%	61%	49%	37%
No	60%	55%	56%	64%	59%	63%	53%	59%	57%	68%	39%	50%	62%
				N.S.				$0.02 > p > 0.01$				$0.02 > p > 0.01$	
Hand Comfort?													
Comfortably warm	21%	13%	20%	28%	23%	26%	12%	22%	19%	33%	13%	24%	22%
Comfortable	35%	29%	38%	29%	40%	44%	31%	35%	37%	39%	18%	24%	37%
Comfortably cool	21%	26%	18%	22%	22%	21%	17%	24%	27%	20%	9%	17%	21%
Too cool	15%	26%	17%	16%	12%	5%	31%	16%	13%	3%	50%	24%	15%
Much too cool	4%	5%	5%	3%	1%	3%	7%	2%	2%	3%	11%	4%	3%
				$p < 0.001$				$p < 0.001$				$0.05 > p > 0.025$	

* This question was asked during the morning interview.

5.5. There is a significant association between the responses to this question and urine temperature levels. There is also a clear and logical trend for living-room temperatures. Thus for morning temperatures, 38% of those with temperatures below 14°C stated that their hands were 'too cool' or 'much too cool' compared to only 6% of those with temperatures of 18°C or above. The answers to this question do relate closely to bedroom temperatures. Thirty-one per cent of those in the below 8°C group were 'too cool' or 'much too cool' compared to only 8% in the 16°C and above group.

General body comfort

We asked those in our sample: 'on the whole how warm or how cool are you feeling at the moment?' The comfort gradings for the different temperature groups are shown in Table 5.6. (No one felt 'much too warm' and only three persons were 'too warm'. These categories are not shown in the table.) There was no significant difference in general body comfort between the two urine temperature groups. About three-quarters of both groups felt either 'comfortable' or 'warm'. However there is a significant association between comfort gradings and living-room temperatures. Twenty-one per cent of those with morning temperatures below 14°C reported being either 'too cool' or 'much too cool' compared to only 7% of those in the 18°C or above group. And as many as 41% of those in the lowest living-room temperature category in both the morning and evening were 'too cool' or 'much too cool' compared to only 11% of the sample as a whole. For bedroom temperatures 18% in the coldest category (below 8°C) felt 'too cool' or 'much too cool' compared to only 4% of the 'warmest' category (16°C and above).

Preference for warmth

Another question – and one with important implications for the prevention of hypothermia – concerned the elderly's preference for warmth. We asked whether our respondents would prefer to be warmer or cooler, with a choice from a five-point scale. (No one wished to be 'very much cooler' and only five 'slightly cooler'. Only the main categories are shown in the table.) As Table 5.7 shows, 7% of the sample would prefer to be 'very much warmer' and a further 21% 'slightly warmer'. There is no statistically significant association between morning urine temperatures and preferences for warmth. However the trend is in the direction one would have expected for living-room and bedroom temperatures. For example 13% of those in the coldest bedrooms (<8) preferred to be 'very much warmer' against only 3% of old people in the warmest bedrooms

Table 5.6

Body Comfort by Room and Urine Temperatures

| | Total | Minimum Bedroom Temperature | | | | | Morning Living-room Temperature | | | | Cold A.M. and P.M. | Urine Temperature A.M. | |
		<8	8<10	10<12	12<16	16+	0–13	14–15	16–17	18+		Under 35.5	36.0+
Total:	1,020	136	203	269	251	73	242	274	228	237	56	98	699
Body Comfort?													
Comfortably warm	27%	22%	26%	30%	26%	36%	19%	31%	26%	33%	20%	23%	27%
Comfortable	49%	42%	48%	49%	56%	51%	45%	46%	57%	51%	27%	47%	50%
Comfortably cool	10%	18%	8%	10%	7%	8%	14%	13%	7%	6%	13%	10%	9%
Too cool	9%	15%	11%	7%	9%	3%	15%	8%	7%	7%	30%	14%	9%
Much too cool	2%	3%	3%	2%	*%	1%	6%	1%	1%	*%	11%	1%	2%
				0.01>p>0.001					p<0.001				N.S.

* This question was asked during the morning interview.

Table 5.7   Preference for Warmth by Room and Urine Temperatures

	Total	Minimum Bedroom Temperature					Morning Living-room Temperature				Cold A.M. and P.M.	Urine Temperature A.M.	
		<8	8<10	10<12	12<16	16+	0–13	14–15	16–17	18+		Under 35.5	36.0+
Total:	1,020	136	203	269	251	73	242	274	228	237	56	98	699
Preference A.M.?													
Very much warmer	7%	13%	9%	4%	5%	3%	13%	5%	4%	4%	23%	11%	6%
Slightly warmer	21%	28%	25%	21%	17%	18%	30%	24%	19%	14%	34%	24%	22%
No change	68%	58%	63%	72%	75%	78%	55%	68%	74%	80%	41%	59%	70%
				p<0.001					p<0.001			N.S.	

No one reported a preference to be 'very much cooler' and only 5 wished to be 'slightly cooler'. Three persons 'did not know'.

(16+) and 80% of those with living-room temperatures of 18°C or above wanted 'no change' against only 55% of those with temperatures below 14°C. Again, 57% of those in the coldest living-rooms in both the evening and morning preferred to be 'very much' or 'slightly' warmer compared to only 28% of the whole sample. But of far greater importance than these statistically significant relationships is the fact that large numbers of the elderly preferred 'no change' despite their living in cold conditions.

Perceptions of the cold

A summary of some of the most interesting responses to the 'comfort' questions is presented in Figure 5.6 and Table A.7 shows the statistical significance of the data. What do these findings tell us about old people's perceptions of the cold? Do they support the view that those at risk from cold conditions might not be aware of their situation and will therefore not seek help? Before drawing together some conclusions from our findings, it

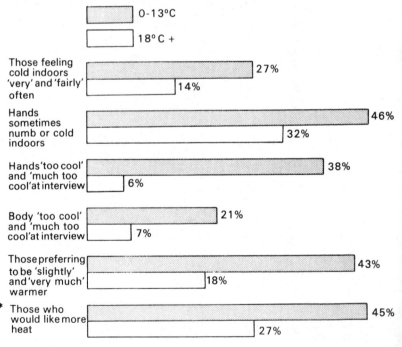

* These data are from table 6.9 (chapter 6)

Figure 5.6 Percentages in Coldest and Warmest Living-rooms for 'Comfort Questions'.

is important to point to the limitations of this kind of data. Our results depend on subjective assessments by each individual and therefore need to be carefully interpreted.

In general it is the case that those with low body temperatures – the 'at risk' group – are more likely than others to report that they often feel cold indoors, have cold hands, and prefer more warmth. Similarly those living in the coldest rooms are generally more likely to be cold and want greater warmth. Thus questions of this kind are useful in a broad way by indicating those with problems of cold housing. Yet they have serious limitations. As we have seen large proportions of both the 'at risk' and of those in the coldest housing report thay they do *not* often feel cold indoors, that their hands do *not* get cold, that they would *not* prefer to be warmer and so on. Why is this? As we said earlier we need to interpret the survey results cautiously. Our results might reflect not so much a person's failure to feel the cold, but rather an unwillingness to report, or admit to, feeling cold and preferring to be warmer. This might be due to pride, independence or a general reluctance to complain.

In practice there will be different explanations of the elderly's seeming acceptance of the cold. It is likely that the elderly's toleration of the cold is higher than, say, that of young office workers, students or many non-pensioner households. These groups are used to – and expect – higher standards (although, physiologically, they can tolerate the cold better than the old). There will be many who suffer from the cold, but will not complain or seek help for the reasons of pride we have mentioned. Others – probably a relatively small group – may eventually fail to feel the cold as their body temperatures fall during cold periods. This may well account for the answers given to our questions by some of our 'at risk' group. Whatever the reasons might be these findings offer no encouragement to medical practitioners and social service staff concerned with the identification and prevention of hypothermia.

Living Alone and Risk

The fact that there was no statistically significant relationship between living alone and low urine temperatures has been briefly noted. However this finding calls for some discussion. It will come as a surprise to those who equate living alone with loneliness and social isolation and consequently regard this group of old people as being especially liable to suffer the effects of cold conditions. In order to explore this hypothesis about hypothermia we asked a number of questions about the position of those living alone and it is worth while briefly to report some of our results.

How do those living alone spend their time? We asked whether they had done certain things 'yesterday'. The results are summarized in Table A.8. In general this presents a picture of an active old age for those living alone. Half of the group had been for a walk and a similar proportion had been shopping. Forty three per cent had met friends outside of their homes and 30 per cent had visited friends or relatives. As many as 57 per cent had had visitors. Three-quarters of the sample had watched television and 69 per cent had listened to the radio. Of course this only presents a snap-shot view, but it does not lend any support to those who regard old age in general as an inactive and unhappy period of life, full of misery and sorrow. Rather it suggests that a good number of those who live alone lead full and positive lives.

These findings however only indicate a broad picture and there are some elderly people living alone who can properly be termed socially isolated (see the evidence presented in Chapter 2). Our own survey results do not enable us to estimate the number that might be termed socially isolated nor to pinpoint the specific causes of such isolation. Nevertheless various points can be made. Regular contact with, and help and support from, children is obviously of importance to the old. We asked those in our sample when they had last seen any of their children. The replies show that very large proportions of the elderly had seen a child on the day of the interview or very recently. However a small minority had not seen their children for some time. The detailed findings are 'today': 49 per cent; 'yesterday': 15 per cent; 'last week': 20 per cent; 'last month': 9 per cent; 'last year' (i.e. 1971, the survey being carried out in January – March 1972): 6 per cent; and 'before January 1971': 2 per cent.

Of course not all old people have children. In fact 27 per cent* of our sample did not have any (10 per cent being single; 15 per cent reporting having had no children; and 2 per cent whose children were dead). Our results would also suggest that a minority of those living alone are relatively isolated. We asked those without visitors 'yesterday' whether they had had visitors during the last 7 days. Forty two per cent of this group had not had visitors during this period, which represents 18 per cent of all of those who were living alone. Such figures do suggest problems, for while those living alone were no more likely to have low body temperatures than those living with others, they are more 'at risk' in a different sense. An old person suffering from the effects of the cold (and a lowering of deep body temperature) stands a chance of this being noted by others in the household. For those who are living alone – particularly the isolated –

---

*This proportion is broadly similar to the estimate of the DHSS: 'probably 25 per cent of all elderly people have no children to assist them in time of need', DHSS. *Conference on the Elderly, 26 July 1977*, **Background Paper**, para 4.

hypothermia may develop without help being available. And, in the extreme case of an elderly person who has no children and receives few visitors, an accident in the home, which leaves the old person unable to attract attention, may result in tragedy.

Conclusion

Given the lack of association between room and inner body temperatures, we did not expect to find significant associations between low body temperatures and those socio-economic factors that might directly bear on the level of room temperatures. The results bear out the expectation and the most noticeable exceptions can be regarded as 'trigger' factors that are strongly associated with the failure of some old people to maintain deep body temperature homeostasis in a cold environment. Age is the most obvious of these factors, but we would warn against overstating its importance – many younger pensioners are also 'at risk'. Although poverty is not directly linked with low deep body temperatures, the receipt of supplementary benefit is. This is an intriguing finding and cannot simply be explained by the greater age of benefit recipients. We argued that the receipt of benefits is an indicator of general deprivation. Our evidence shows that the combination of a declining physiology and the most deprived social circumstances greatly increase the risk of an old person becoming hypothermic. We found two factors that were significantly associated with low body temperatures which might be reasonably expected to have an 'immediate' influence on them. Body weight would appear to have an influence on deep body temperature which is independent of age, but might also, in part, explain the importance of age (as more of the very aged are underweight). The other factor is the possession of electric blankets which would appear to be an important preventive measure.

The results reported in this chapter offer no simple answers to those concerned with identifying and helping those most 'at risk' from the cold. Nevertheless certain factors have been identified that appear to be of importance and the implications of these findings are discussed in the final chapter. However there is no evidence to suggest that the cold elderly will identify themselves as such, still less ask for the help that some of them so desperately need.

Results

Chapter 6 Cold Homes and Social Conditions

The last chapter was concerned with body temperatures and the social circumstances of those 'at risk'. Here we shift attention to the home environment and cold conditions. Obviously this directly relates to the danger of hypothermia. For although there is no correlation between room and deep body temperatures – and while those in the coldest conditions do not necessarily have low body temperatures – it is undoubtedly the case that a minority of those in cold homes become 'at risk' of developing hypothermia. A study of the social circumstances in which low room temperatures are likely to be found is therefore important because of this link with hypothermia. But, as we have said before, we were also interested in cold housing as a social problem in its own right and not just because of its link with physical health.

Demographic and Household Circumstances

In exploring the particular social circumstances that are associated with cold homes, an obvious starting point is demographic and household characteristics. Are there any major groups, such as the single or those living alone, who are likely to be in the coldest homes? In fact, as Table A.9 shows, an analysis of such factors by room temperatures offers no simple short-cuts to identifying the cold elderly. There is no difference between the sexes, nor does marital status seem to be important. Whilst the single were over-represented in the coldest living-rooms (16% of those in the below 14°C group compared to only 8% in the 18°C+ group) this pattern is not reflected for bedrooms. Neither does household composition offer any quick means of identifying the cold elderly. Although those living alone do appear to be in colder living rooms than others, the differences do not reach the level of significance.

How does age relate to room temperatures? Do the very aged live in colder homes than younger pensioners? Again there is no obvious pattern and the evidence in Table A.10 shows that a fair cross-section of all elderly age groups live in the coldest conditions. As we explained in the last

Table 6.1

Tenure of Housing by Minimum Bedroom and Living-room Temperatures

	Total	Minimum Bedroom Temperatures					A.M. Living-room Temperatures				Cold A.M. and P.M.
		<8	8<10	10<12	12<16	16+	0–13	14–15	16–17	18+	
Total	1,020	136	203	269	251	73	242	274	228	237	56
Tenure											
Owner-occupied	39%	51%	35%	36%	43%	38%	40%	35%	43%	39%	43%
Rented from local authority	38%	22%	35%	41%	41%	41%	41%	38%	29%	44%	39%
Rented from housing association	3%	1%	2%	1%	2%	7%	3%	1%	1%	4%	4%
Privately rented — Furnished	1%	1%	—	1%	*%	1%	1%	1%	2%	—	4%
Privately rented— Unfurnished	19%	24%	27%	19%	13%	12%	14%	24%	25%	12%	11%
Other	1%	—	1%	1%	*%	—	*%	—	—	—	—
		p<0.001					N.S.				

chapter the over-representation of the very aged in our 'at risk' group cannot simply be explained in terms of environmental temperatures.

Housing

Housing was always likely to be a crucial aspect of the problem of the cold elderly. Equally, better housing policies and management are a major element in the prevention of hypothermia in particular and cold conditions in general.

We have already established in Chapter 5 that there is no direct association between low body temperatures and housing type, tenure, or lack of amenities. The purpose of this section is to explore whether particular housing circumstances are likely to be associated with cold living conditions.

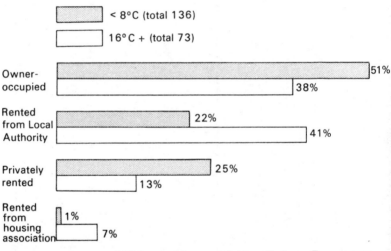

Figure 6.1 Percentages of Highest and Lowest Minimum Bedroom Temperature Levels by Tenure.

Tenure

To what extent does the *tenure* of a dwelling have an association with room temperature? Table 6.1 presents data on both living-room and minimum bedroom temperatures and Figure 6.1 illustrates the main findings. It shows that for living-rooms there is no discernible difference between tenures. The figures for bedrooms tell a different story however. It would appear that, in general, local authority tenants are more likely to have warmer bedrooms at night than either owner-occupiers or private tenants. Thus whereas only 22% of those with minimum bedroom temperatures below 8°C lived in council accommodation, the figure for those in the 16°C+ group was 41%. These results to some extent reflect the data on house type given later, for many of the purpose-built flats are likely to be local-authority owned.

Amenities

The relationship between 'bad' housing and room temperature levels has also been tested. An inadequate house was clearly likely to be an inefficient thermal unit. It was obviously not possible, however, in a large study such as this to survey each house to ascertain its thermal adequacy. Some short-cut measure of bad housing was necessary. Housing that lacks certain basic amenities is used here to represent 'bad' housing. This would seem to be a reasonable indicator. For example, according to the 1971 National House Condition Survey, 80% of all unfit dwellings in England and Wales lacked one or more of the basic amenities. The proportion for fit dwellings was only 12%[1].

Accordingly we asked those in our sample whether or not they had exclusive use of certain basic amenities, and an analysis of these results by temperature is given in Table 6.2. From this it is clear that there is no general association between living-room temperatures and the possession of amenities, although it is striking that 41% of the 'cold A.M. and P.M.' living-room group lacked exclusive use of amenities. However, again the results for bedrooms show a different picture. Here there is a direct relationship between low minimum temperatures and the lack of exclusive use of basic amenities. For example, 38% of the group with temperatures below 8°C lacked exclusive use of amenities, compared to 16% of those in the 16°C and above group.

House type

From the analysis of living-room temperatures by type of house given in Table 6.3 no straightforward pattern emerges. It might have been expected that those house-types that are likely to be relatively spacious − e.g. detached houses − would be colder than those that are smaller. This is not the case. Nevertheless, it is noticeable that the one-fifth of our sample who lived in purpose-built flats fared relatively well. Although some of this accommodation was very cold − accounting for 16% of all accommodation with morning temperatures below 14°C − it did make up almost one-third (31%) of all accommodation with temperatures of 18°C or over. It would also seem that those in semi-detached housing were generally experiencing lower living-room temperature levels in the morning.

Table 6.2   Possession of Amenities by Minimum Bedroom and Living-room Temperatures

	Total	Minimum Bedroom Temperatures					A.M. Living-room Temperatures				
		<8	8<10	10<12	12<16	16+	0–13	14–15	16–17	18+	Cold A.M. and P.M.
Total	1,020	136	203	269	251	73	242	274	228	237	56
*Use of Amenities**											
Exclusive Use	70%	63%	68%	70%	74%	84%	67%	71%	69%	71%	59%
Lack of Exclusive Use	30%	38%	32%	30%	26%	16%	33%	29%	31%	29%	41%
		0.02>p>0.1					N.S.				

* Fixed bath; kitchen sink; W.C. indoors or attached to house; hot water at bath, kitchen sink and hand-basin.

Table 6.3 Type of Accommodation by Minimum Bedroom and Living-room Temperatures

| | Total | Minimum Bedroom Temperatures | | | | | A.M. Living-room Temperatures | | | | |
		<8	8<10	10<12	12<16	16+	0–13	14–15	16–17	18+	Cold A.M. and P.M.
Total	1,020	136	203	269	251	73	242	274	228	237	56
Type of Accommodation											
Detached	12%	14%	12%	11%	10%	12%	12%	8%	14%	11%	11%
Semi-detached	27%	32%	27%	28%	30%	30%	31%	35%	20%	22%	34%
Terraced	33%	45%	40%	38%	26%	18%	36%	35%	38%	26%	34%
Part house/rooms	4%	4%	4%	4%	6%	1%	3%	3%	7%	4%	4%
Purpose-built flat/maisonette	20%	4%	15%	18%	25%	37%	16%	15%	17%	31%	14%
Converted flat/maisonette	2%	1%	2%	2%	3%	—	1%	3%	3%	1%	2%
Bed-sitter	2%	—	—	—	1%	1%	*%	1%	2%	3%	—
				p<0.001					p<0.001		

In addition 2 respondents lived in 'other' accommodation.

An analysis by minimum bedroom temperatures shows a similar picture in respect of terraced houses. Whereas 45% of all dwellings with bedroom temperatures below 8°C were terraced, this type of housing represented only 18% of houses with bedroom temperatures of 16°C or over. Again, those in purpose-built flats fared substantially better. Only 4% of those with bedroom temperatures below 8°C lived in this type of housing compared to 37% of those with temperatures of 16°C or over.

The most striking fact to emerge from Table 6.3, however, is that living-room temperatures in the mornings and minimum bedroom temperatures were generally low whatever the type of housing. So, while the type of housing an elderly person occupies does make a difference to the warmth of the house, not one of the main house-type categories in the sample had average temperatures at the recommended levels.

Number of bedrooms

As stated earlier, one reason for considering temperature levels according to house type was due to the association between the latter and house size. A more direct indicator of this is the number of bedrooms. However as can be seen from Table A.11 an analysis by living-room temperatures reveals no obvious correlation between number of bedrooms and cold conditions. On reflection this is perhaps not surprising. Some of the elderly living in relatively large accommodation will be sharing it with others and it is therefore more likely to be kept warm. It also seems reasonable to assume that in general (and there are important exceptions) those living in larger accommodation will be relatively better off than those in smaller accommodation and consequently relatively in a better position to heat their homes.

It is perhaps when bedrooms are not being used that heating problems may occur as this might indicate general under-occupation and, in some cases, a problem of too little income with which to heat too large a space. Table A.11 presents the results of a simple analysis based on answers to our question: 'Are there any of these (bedrooms) you seldom use?' This suggests that those having one or more bedrooms not in use were more likely to have lower living-room temperatures. Fifty-two per cent of those with temperatures below 14°C were in this category compared to 38% with temperatures at or above 18°C.

Satisfaction with housing

Are those living in cold conditions more likely to be dissatisfied with their housing than others? Table 6.4 suggests that this is the case. Thus,

Table 6.4   *Satisfaction with Accommodation by Minimum Bedroom and Living-room Temperatures*

		Minimum Bedroom Temperatures					A.M. Living-room Temperatures				
	Total	<8	8<10	10<12	12<16	16+	0–13	14–15	16–17	18+	Cold A.M. and P.M.
Total	1,020	136	203	269	251	73	242	274	228	237	56
Satisfaction with Accommodation											
Completely satisfied	70%	61%	62%	72%	80%	81%	60%	68%	73%	76%	48%
Fairly satisfied	19%	26%	20%	18%	12%	11%	21%	22%	18%	16%	30%
Neither satisfied nor dissatisfied	2%	4%	3%	2%	*%	—	3%	3%	1%	1%	2%
Rather dissatisfied	6%	6%	11%	4%	6%	5%	10%	5%	6%	5%	13%
Completely dissatisfied	3%	2%	4%	3%	2%	3%	5%	3%	2%	2%	7%
				p<0.001					0.025>p>0.01		

whereas 60% of those with morning living-room temperatures below 14°C reported being completely satisfied with their accommodation, the proportion rose to 76% of those with temperatures of 18°C or above. A similar result is shown from the analysis by minimum bedroom temperatures. It is also interesting that only half (48%) of the 'cold A.M. and P.M.' group were completely satisfied and 20% were 'rather' or 'completely' dis-

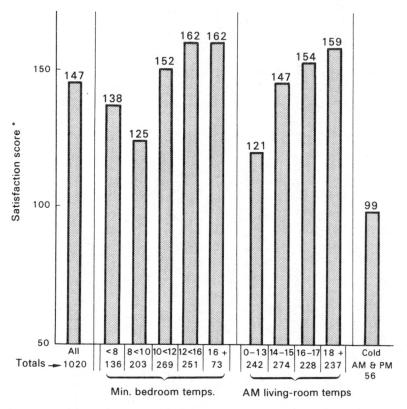

*Score calculated:– completely satisfied + 2, fairly satisfied + 1, rather dissatisfied –1, completely dissatisfied –2, neither satisfied nor dissatisfied 0.

Figure 6.2 Satisfaction with Accommodation by Minimum Bedroom and A.M. Living-room Temperatures.

satisfied. Figure 6.2 presents the data differently by 'scoring' responses to this question. This graphically illustrates the effect of cold rooms on satisfaction with housing. Perhaps of most significance however is the fact that the vast majority of all groups – including those in the coldest conditions – were 'satisfied', or at least 'fairly satisfied' with their accommodation. Thus 87% of those in the coldest bedrooms (below 8°C) reported being 'satisfied'.

Heating

Heating methods are obviously likely to be one of the most important factors that determine temperature levels. Having established that there is *no* clear association between room temperatures and the urine temperatures of the elderly, a correlation between the latter and heating methods is not to be expected. But one would reasonably expect an association between room temperatures and heating methods. However, before considering temperature levels, it is useful to look at the heating methods used by Britain's elderly. A wide variety of types of heating are used and any single household is very likely to possess more than one appliance. In fact while 20% of the sample (207 persons) had only one 'appliance'; 46% (471) had two; 22% (220) three; 6% (57) four; 3% (35) five; and 2% (17) had six or more. A very disturbing finding was that 13 old people (1%) reported having no heating appliances at all. Altogether 24% of the sample had central heating. More detailed information about heating types is given in Table 6.5. It can be seen that electric was the most common form of central heating and was found in 10% of all households. Very large proportions of the sample had 'conventional' appliances. The most 'popular' were coal fires (61%) and electric radiant heaters (57%).

The usage of heating appliances depended a great deal on the type in question. In particular a distinction can be made between central heating and other forms of heating. The vast majority of respondents with central heating (from 88% – 96% according to type) reported that they used their heating 'regularly'. We also asked 'On average in winter how many hours a day do you use it?' The great majority of those with central heating reported using it for a large number of hours – the majority over thirteen hours a day.

The pattern of usage varied a great deal within the non-central heating category. While 89% of those with solid fuel used their fires 'regularly', the proportions for other types ranged from 81% for gas convectors to 40% for paraffin radiant. In interpreting these and later figures it is important to bear in mind that the owner of one type of heating may not be using an appliance 'regularly' or even 'sometimes' because he is using other forms of heating (possibly central heating) regularly. Many appliances will be for 'emergencies' or only occasional use. The reported use of 'conventional' appliances is generally confirmed by the data on the number of hours for which appliances are used on average.

Table 6.5

Heating: Methods and Amount of Use

Type	No.	% of Total	Regularity of Use as % of Heating Type			Hours used 'on average in winter' as % of Heating Type			
			Regularly	Sometimes	Never	3 or less	4–8	9–13	13+
Central Heating									
Gas	59	6	93	2	—	2	17	27	51
Electric	106	10	88	7	4	6	6	12	74
Coal/smokeless	51	5	94	2	—	—	2	16	78
Oil	28	3	96	4	—	4	4	21	71
Non-Central Heating									
Gas convector	131	13	81	18	2	18	16	27	38
Gas radiant	161	16	77	20	2	21	15	25	38
Electric convector	174	17	51	45	3	51	20	11	13
Electric radiant	577	57	42	52	5	59	21	8	6
Coal/smokeless	621	61	89	7	2	5	10	33	49
Paraffin radiant	48	5	40	40	21	27	25	6	19
Paraffin convector	150	15	53	39	6	34	28	15	17
Other	21	2	76	19	5	29	10	14	43
No heating	13	1							

The effect of central heating

What type of association is there between heating types and temperature levels? In particular, does central heating make a significant difference to the heating standards achieved? Table 6.6 compares the room temperatures of those with and without central heating and some of the main

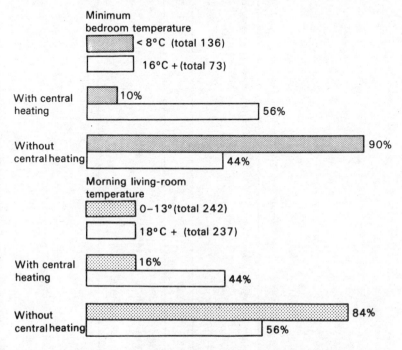

Figure 6.3 Percentages of Highest and Lowest Room Temperature Groups by Central Heating.

results are illustrated in Figure 6.3. There is a statistically significant association between the possession of central heating and living-room temperatures. Those with higher room temperatures were more likely to possess central heating. For morning living-rooms only 16% of those with temperatures below 14°C had central heating, while the proportion is 44% for the 18°C and above group. The evidence for minimum bedroom temperatures is even more clear-cut. For example, only 10% of the below 8°C group had central heating compared to 56% of the 16°C and above group. And it is particularly significant that 96% of the group with the coldest living-rooms in both the morning and evening did not have central heating. The finding that those with central heating are living in warmer homes than others may seem to be an unexceptional – indeed obvious – conclusion.

Table 6.6

Central Heating by Room Temperature Levels

	Total	Minimum Bedroom Temperatures					A.M. Living-room Temperatures				
		<8	8<10	10<12	12<16	16+	0–13	14–15	16–17	18+	Cold A.M. and P.M.
Total	1,020	136	203	269	251	73	242	274	228	237	56
Central Heating	23%	10%	16%	18%	35%	56%	16%	15%	21%	44%	4%
No Central Heating	77%	90%	84%	82%	65%	44%	84%	85%	79%	56%	96%
				p<0.001					p<0.001		

However, it is more interesting than it appears. Many of those concerned about the welfare of the elderly have worried that sophisticated central heating systems may not always keep old people warmer because they are complex, because they are looked upon suspiciously and because of the expense. Consequently they may not be used. All of these problems are no doubt valid in certain cases and central heating certainly has to be simple and relatively inexpensive in order to be really effective. However, our findings suggest that over the country as a whole – at least during the survey period – central heating was producing higher room temperatures for the elderly.

Heating in the bedroom

It is often argued that the problem of the cold elderly stems not so much (or not only) from inadequate heating systems or from low incomes, but rather from a failure to use the heating that is available, particularly in the bedroom.

We therefore asked those taking part in the survey whether they heated the room that they 'sleep in'. Table 6.7 shows the answers to this question and analyses them by temperature levels. It is interesting to see that almost half (47%) of the sample did not heat the room they slept in.* This can probably be put down to a number of factors which include the traditional British dislike of heating bedrooms (and, indeed, a tendency towards opening windows, even on very cold nights); expense; perhaps the greater difficulty of providing heat in bedrooms; and fears about having a fire unattended. Ten per cent of the sample reported heating their 'sleeping' rooms 'all night', while 29% heated them 'just before going to bed'.

How do bedroom heating practices affect temperature levels? Our results suggest that there is a logical, important, but not particularly dramatic effect. For example, only 2% of those with minimum bedroom temperatures below 8°C heated their bedroom 'all night', whereas 25% of the 16°C and above group did. However, although the majority (59%) in the coldest bedrooms (below 8°C) did not heat their bedrooms, the figure was as high as 42% for those in the warmest.

A correlation between living-room temperatures and the heating of 'bedrooms' might be expected, particularly for morning temperatures. Thus, for example, only 6% of those with morning living-room temperatures below 14°C heated their 'bedroom' all night compared to 18% of those with temperatures of 18°C or above. It is also interesting to note that those with very cold living-room temperatures in both the morning and

*See Chapter 9 for information on bedroom heating habits in the forties and fifties.

Table 6.7

Heating of Bedrooms by Room Temperature Levels

	Total	Minimum Bedroom Temperatures					A.M. Living-room Temperatures				
		<8	8<10	10<12	12<16	16+	0–13	14–15	16–17	18+	Cold A.M. and P.M.
Total	1,020	136	203	269	251	73	242	274	228	237	56
Bedroom Heated											
All night	10%	2%	4%	6%	16%	25%	6%	5%	10%	18%	2%
Just before going to bed	29%	32%	32%	29%	31%	23%	27%	27%	32%	29%	16%
Not at all	47%	59%	53%	53%	43%	42%	52%	51%	46%	40%	63%
				p<0.001					p<0.001		

(In addition to the responses listed above, 6% had bed-sitting rooms, slept in the living-room or heated their bedroom all day and a further 8% of the sample gave other answers to this question, e.g. bedroom heated in morning and evening; only in very cold weather.)

afternoon were much more likely than others not to heat their bedrooms, accounting for 63% of this group.

There is, not surprisingly, a close connection between the heating of bedrooms and the type of heating in the home. Thus, whereas 29% of those with central heating heated their bedroom 'all night', 30% 'just before going to bed' and 29% 'not at all', the proportions for those without central heating were 4%, 29% and 53% respectively. These findings show the greater ease with which bedrooms can be kept warm at night if central heating is available and confirm the importance of central heating in the fight against cold conditions.

Poverty and Heating Costs

In Chapter 5 we explored the implications of the association between low deep body temperatures and receipt of supplementary benefits. The seemingly obvious explanation that poverty was the key factor is, in fact, not supported by the evidence about supplementary benefits and room temperatures (Table A.2) and income levels and temperatures (Table A.3). It is useful at this stage to analyse the poverty question a little more carefully.

What is meant by poverty in old age? In practice most analysts are willing to accept the supplementary benefit level (or some level based on it) as a working definition. For this reason we considered it worth while to analyse temperature data by the receipt or non-receipt of benefit. However, given a large degree of non take-up, this is only a crude approximation of the division between the poor and non-poor elderly. We therefore also presented data analysed by income categories and on this basis were able to investigate the 'poverty factor' further. But even this rather more sophisticated analysis has drawbacks, particularly when considering subjects such as heating and warmth. In the brief review of the financial circumstances of the elderly in Chapter 2 we argued that, compared to the rest of the population, the elderly were generally a relatively poor group in society. This is confirmed by our own data on incomes. But for the purpose of analysis we split incomes into three categories (See Table A.3). Thus, for single persons, the 'poor' category was up to £7.50 weekly income, the middle group, £7.50–£10.50 and the top group, more than £10.50. But is there not a danger of such categorization concealing more than it reveals? Obviously the person who receives £8 a week is usually better off than the one who only gets £6. But what if the former lives in a large house which is difficult to heat and the latter in a purpose-built, centrally heated flat?

The effect of financial hardship on heating is not solely a product of income levels, but also depends on the adequacy of income to cope with individual needs and circumstances. It is not just the statistically (and arbitrarily) defined poorest who face problems, but also the poor and the hard-pressed. For these reasons it is difficult to demonstrate adequately the relationship between income and room temperature levels – there are too many intervening variables – and, as we have seen, in the case of low urine temperatures, other factors will be important.

Heating costs

An analysis of heating costs is one direct way of considering the importance of poverty for our explanation of cold conditions. The cost of heating is a major problem for many of the elderly and, in many cases, is likely to be a direct cause of cold housing. It is also a problem that has certainly increased in importance since the time of our survey. However, the accurate recording of weekly, monthly and annual heating costs is difficult and complex. Whereas in some cases it might be relatively straightforward – where, say, central heating only is used – in many other cases estimating heating costs will be a major exercise. For example, one household might use gas and electric fires, paraffin heaters and solid fuel. Some bills will be paid monthly or quarterly while other fuels will be paid for at the time of purchase or delivery. The collection of such expenditure data was outside the scope of our survey approach and we rejected short-cuts – such as householder's estimates – as likely to be unreliable. The Family Expenditure Survey, however, gives very useful information about spending on heating – see Chapter 2 – and it is clear from this that the poorest elderly have next to no room for manoeuvre in the weekly balancing act between adequate nutrition, the purchase of household necessities and reasonable warmth.

While unable to collect data on heating costs we did ask a simple question about attitudes to the expense of heating. As can be seen from Table 6.8 only 2% found it 'rather cheap' and only 27% 'reasonable'. Two-thirds of our elderly respondents found it 'rather expensive'. This general consensus of opinion about the cost of heating is probably the most important point to emerge from the table. But for living-room temperatures it also shows an association between views on the cost of heating and the temperature levels that were actually being achieved. The pattern is also broadly in the expected direction for bedroom temperatures. Those who were living in colder conditions were more likely to find their heating expensive.

Table 6.8

Views about Cost of Heating by Room Temperatures

	Total	Minimum Bedroom Temperatures					A.M. Living-room Temperatures				
		<8	8<10	10<12	12<16	16+	0–13	14–15	15–16	18+	Cold A.M. and P.M.
Total	1,020	136	203	269	251	73	242	274	228	237	56
Expense of Heating											
1. Rather cheap	2%	1%	1%	4%	2%	1%	2%	3%	1%	3%	2%
2. Reasonable	27%	25%	20%	29%	27%	36%	19%	24%	29%	35%	16%
3. Rather expensive	67%	69%	76%	64%	66%	56%	74%	71%	63%	57%	79%
4. Don't know	4%	5%	3%	2%	5%	5%	4%	2%	6%	5%	4%
				0.025>p>0.01					0.01>p>0.001		

More heat in the home?

We also asked our sample whether they would 'generally like to have more heat in the home?' As can be seen from Table 6.9 37% replied 'yes' to this question and 61% 'no'. Given the evidence presented earlier that the majority of the elderly live in homes that are colder than is desirable this response may seem surprising (but it is in line with the responses to other attitudinal questions reported in Chapter 5). It is likely, however, that the

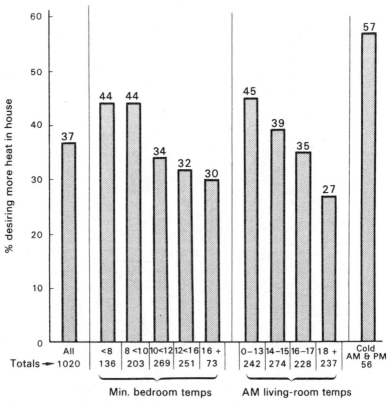

Figure 6.4 Attitude to having Heat in House by Room Temperature.

finding that a large proportion of old people profess no desire for more heat in their homes reflects a variety of factors including, on the one hand, an habitual tolerance of temperatures that younger age-groups would find too low for comfort and, on the other, a worry about the expense of any additional heating.

Figure 6.4 illustrates the association between room temperature and the

Table 6.9

Attitude to Having More Heat in House by Room Temperatures

	Total	Minimum Bedroom Temperatures					A.M. Living-room Temperatures				Cold A.M. and P.M.
		<8	8<10	10<12	12<16	16+	0–13	14–15	16–17	18+	
Total	1,020	136	203	269	251	73	242	274	228	237	56
More Heat in House?											
1. Yes	37%	44%	44%	34%	32%	30%	45%	39%	35%	27%	57%
2. No	61%	54%	55%	64%	66%	68%	52%	60%	64%	71%	41%
3. Don't know	2%	2%	1%	2%	2%	1%	3%	1%	1%	1%	2%
				0.02>p>0.01					p<0.001		

desire for more heat. Responses to this question are significantly associated with environmental temperatures. Forty-five per cent of those with morning living-room temperatures at or below 13°C expressed a wish for more heating compared to 27% of those with temperatures of 18°C or above. There is a similar trend for minimum bedroom temperatures. And, not surprisingly, 57% of those in the coldest living-rooms, both morning and evening, would have liked more heat in the house. Those who stated that they would like more heat in the house were asked 'Why do you not have more heating?' Eighty-eight per cent gave answers such as 'too expensive' or 'can't afford more' or other reasons concerning the cost of heating. These responses − together with those to the question about the expense of heating − demonstrate that the cost of heating was preventing many of Britain's elderly from having warmer homes. This conclusion is in line with the findings of the Supplementary Benefits Commission's Inspectorate that, in the winter of 1975/76, many supplementary pensioners were unduly restricting their heating because of worries about cost[2].

Those in receipt of supplementary pension (some 34% of the sample) were asked 'Do you receive a special fuel allowance as part of your supplementary pension? Only 3% replied that they did. Now in fact a much higher proportion of our sample must have been receiving a fuel allowance at this time (1972). This lack of knowledge is not as surprising as it may at first appear. An old person does not always have to claim an extra addition for fuel (in a way comparable to the claiming of a supplementary benefit itself) and many old people may be awarded an addition without their being at all clear about it. All they may know is that they get so much 'supplementary' on top of the basic pension.

Supplementary pensioners not claiming to receive a fuel allowance were asked 'Do you know that in certain circumstances old people can get extra money for heating?' As many as 74% replied 'no' to this question. The policy of awarding supplementary benefit heating additions (and the need for more effective publicity for them) is considered in Chapter 7.

Physical mobility

Were the physically incapacitated more likely or less likely to be living in the coldest conditions? From Table A.12 it can be seen that, in fact, there is little difference in temperature levels between those who 'can' and those who 'cannot' get about indoors. Nevertheless, it remains a cause of concern that 10% of those with morning living-room temperatures below 14°C were immobile. This group will obviously find it more difficult than others to keep reasonably warm in such cold conditions.

Contacts with Social and Medical Services

To what extent were the elderly in our sample receiving personal social services, and were our 'at risk' group and those in the coldest homes more or less likely to be the recipients of such services? We asked each of our respondents to name the services they received and the interviewers used a list of services to 'prompt' if necessary. We simplified matters by using the name 'welfare officer' as this was felt to be more meaningful to many of the elderly. We also employed a broad definition of 'services'. We were anxious to establish what service personnel, statutory or voluntary, visited the elderly. We included both formal personal social services and just simple contacts, such as a call from the 'rent man'. We also asked how regularly services were received. The results are presented in Table 6.10 and they are of interest quite apart from any consideration of temperature levels.

The results broadly confirm the findings of the General Household Survey reported in Chapter 2. Each of the main services reaches only small minorities of the elderly. Thus 8% had the services of a domestic or home help, 4% were visited by a 'welfare officer', 4% by health visitors and 3% by 'meals-on-wheels'. However, a larger proportion – 23% – had a contact with the local authority (usually on a fairly regular basis) through the 'rent man'.

For the purposes of analysing the information about social service callers by temperature data, a distinction can be made between the 'welfare' services (i.e. domestic or home help, welfare officer, health visitor and meals-on-wheels) and all 'social service' callers (i.e. all those listed in Table 6.10). The results are presented in Table 6.11. It is interesting to see from this that 15% of the sample received one or more of the 'welfare' services, while 37% received a caller from one or more of the services listed in Table 6.10.

The analysis by temperature shows no clear association between receipt of services and either low urine temperature or cold conditions. In fact, 17% of the 'at risk' group received one or more of the 'welfare' services compared to 13% of the normal group. This difference is not statistically significant. On the one hand therefore, there is no evidence to support one fear, namely that those 'at risk' from the cold might be that section of the aged who are socially isolated, strongly independent and reluctant to accept help from social welfare agents. However, on the other hand, it is not the case that the 'at risk' are significantly more likely to be receiving support than others. Based on this one criterion of cold stress the services are not being directed at all (or even most) of the vulnerable. Nevertheless, that 43% of the 'at risk' received a caller from a social service agency (and

Table 6.10

Visits from Welfare and Other Social Services

	Number Receiving Calls		5 days a week at least		1–4 days each week		Less than once a week but once a month		Less than once a month		Don't know or can't remember	
	No.	% of Total	No.	%	No.	%	No.	%	No.	%	No.	%
Domestic/home help	77	8	15	19	60	78	3	4	—	—	—	—
Welfare officer	46	4	2	4	2	4	6	13	28	61	6	13
Health visitor	48	4	2	4	5	10	5	10	32	67	5	10
Rent man	239	23	1	*	56	23	164	69	15	6	1	*
Meals-on-wheels	27	3	6	22	20	74	1	4	—	—	—	—
Other voluntary organization workers (like Task Force or children from schools)	9	1	1	11	3	33	2	22	2	22	1	11
Chiropodist	56	6	—	—	—	—	10	18	42	75	3	5
Other	26	2	2	8	9	35	11	42	2	8	2	8

Table 6.11

Social Service Callers by Temperatures

| | Total | A.M. Living-room Temperatures | | | | Cold A.M. and P.M. | A.M. Urine Temperature | |
		0–13	14–15	16–17	18+		Under 35.5	36.0+
Total	1,020	242	274	228	237	56	98	699
Any 'Welfare' Caller*	15%	17%	16%	11%	14%	11%	17%	13%
No 'Welfare' Caller	85%	83%	84%	89%	86%	89%	83%	87%
Any Social Services Caller**	37%	40%	45%	32%	32%	34%	43%	36%
No Social Services Caller	63%	60%	55%	68%	68%	66%	57%	64%

The 'Any Welfare' rows are marked N.S. and the 'Any Social Services' rows are marked N.S.

* Domestic/Home Help; Welfare Officer; Health Visitor; Meals-on-wheels.
** All listed in Table 6.10.

37% of the whole sample) is important and has implications for preventive policy which we discuss in our concluding chapter.

We were also interested in how regularly the elderly saw doctors and whether there was any significant differences between the 'at risk' and 'cold' groups and the rest of our sample in this respect. The answers to this question are given in Table 6.12. A substantial proportion of the aged see

Table 6.12

Contact with Doctor by Temperatures

| | Total | A.M. Living-room Temperatures | | | | Cold A.M. and P.M. | A.M. Urine Temperature | |
		0–13	14–15	16–17	18+		Under 35.5	36.0+
Total	1,020	242	274	228	237	56	98	699
When Doctor Last Seen:								
Less than 1 week ago	10%	8%	11%	11%	13%	5%	13%	10%
More than 1 week/1 month	23%	23%	20%	23%	26%	18%	24%	23%
More than 1/3 months	18%	18%	18%	18%	19%	23%	15%	18%
More than 3 months/1 year	19%	21%	19%	18%	17%	13%	19%	18%
More than 1 year ago	25%	24%	30%	24%	23%	27%	24%	25%
Can't remember	4%	6%	3%	6%	2%	14%	3%	4%

their doctors quite frequently. Thus, 10% reported seeing their doctors 'less than one week ago' while a further 23% saw him 'more than one week – but less than one month ago'. However, at the other end of the scale it is perhaps equally interesting that a quarter of the elderly stated that they last saw their doctor 'more than one year ago'.

In seeking this information about contacts with a doctor, we had no firm hypothesis in mind about temperature levels. On the one hand, might it be that the 'at risk' were in regular contact with their GPs because of general health problems? Or, on the other, were they likely to be just the group not obtaining medical help? In fact the results from Table 6.12 do not support either line of thought. Those with low body temperatures had contacts with their GPs that were similar to those of the normal group. However, this means that about a quarter (24%) of those 'at risk' of developing hypothermia – just those who should be urgently seeking medical advice – reported that they had not seen a doctor for more than one year, while a further one fifth (19%) had not seen one for between three months and one year. These findings are very disturbing. It is worth recording, however, that the vast majority (96%) of our sample were able to tell our interviewer the name of their doctor.

Conclusions

The findings presented in this chapter show that there are no short-cuts to the identification of those in the coldest homes in terms of sex, marital status, household composition or age. Regarding housing, council tenants are more likely to have warmer bedrooms, while dwellings lacking basic amenities have colder bedrooms. Purpose-built flats were warmer than other house types and elderly people with one or more bedrooms seldom in use had colder homes. Not surprisingly, those with colder conditions were more dissatisfied with their accommodation, although most of the sample – whatever their room temperatures – reported that they were satisfied with their housing.

Britain's elderly tend to have more than one heating appliance. Less than one-quarter of the sample had central heating, but it was being regularly used and those possessing it had significantly warmer homes than others. Only one in ten of the elderly heated their bedrooms 'all night' and almost a half did not heat them at all.

It is difficult to assess the effect of financial hardship on heating because many other factors are influential. It is also important to remember that most of the elderly are poor, relative to the rest of the population. As expected, most of the elderly found heating expensive and cost was the major reason why those wanting more heat in the house did not have it.

Only small proportions of the aged receive social service callers and there were no significant findings here in relation to temperature levels.

Similarly the 'at risk' and those in the coldest rooms were neither more nor less likely than others to be in contact with their doctors. Nevertheless, the finding that one-quarter of the 'at risk' had not seen a doctor for more than a year is disturbing.

Policy

Chapter 7: Social Security

One of the purposes of the national survey was to explore the relationship between poverty and low temperatures. The picture that emerged from our results (see Chapters 5 and 6) was not entirely clear. While there is an association between the receipt of supplementary benefits and low urine temperature, the latter is not associated with income. Nor are benefit recipients living in colder homes than other pensioners. The greater age of benefit recipients is not the sole explanation. We concluded that the general relative deprivation of supplementary pensioners is a crucial factor. While we must be wary of simple explanations, the greater tendency for benefit recipients to be 'at risk' focuses attention on the supplementary benefits scheme.

The aim of this chapter is to explore the way this part of the social security system attempts to deal with heating costs. It reviews the changing policies of the Supplementary Benefits Commission (SBC) in recent years and concludes by discussing the options for future policy development.

Supplementary Benefits

The financial circumstances of the elderly and social security provisions were briefly described in Chapter 2. We noted that, while the national insurance scheme was originally intended to protect all contributors against the worst effects of loss of earnings, the level of the basic pension has always been – and remains – below the 'poverty line', i.e. the supplementary benefit level (scale rates plus rent). Consequently, a person with only a basic pension and no additional income, or only a small one, will be eligible for supplementary benefit. The supplementary benefit system is therefore a major social welfare institution for the elderly. In December 1976 there were 1,687,000 pensioners claiming supplementary benefit (comprising about 23% of all retired people).[1]

Supplementary benefit is a complex system and particularly that part of it concerned with the exercise of discretion. This chapter is mainly concerned with one aspect of discretion: the granting of exceptional circumstances additions for heating.

Exceptional circumstances additions (ECAs) have become in recent years a major element of supplementary benefits and are particularly important in the case of heating costs. How do such additions relate to the major element of supplementary benefits? What is their purpose? On what grounds are they awarded? Are they effective? Are there alternative approaches? And (more generally) how do they affect the character of supplementary benefits and social security in Britain? These questions and others need to be considered in the context of the recent history of discretionary additions and their relationship to the supplementary benefit system in general.

The decline and rise of discretion

The award of ECAs has been subject to a number of changes in the past ten years and it is useful briefly to trace these and the shifting relationship between discretion and other parts of the supplementary benefit system. At the time of our 1972 National Survey the weekly amount of benefit could be made up of four elements: (1) the scale rates; (2) rent and rates; (3) a long-term addition (awarded to virtually all supplementary pensioners); and (4) exceptional circumstances additions (awarded to only a minority of pensioners).

The scale rates

A supplementary pensioner receives a basic amount of money that is intended to bring income up to a minimum level sufficient to meet needs. Thus, according to the *Supplementary Benefits Handbook:*

> The scale rates are regarded as covering all normal needs which can be foreseen, including food, fuel and light, the normal repair and replacement of clothing, household sundries (but not major items of bedding and furnishing) and provision for amenities such as newspapers, entertainments and radio and television licences ... What the scale rates provide is an amount for people to meet all ordinary living expenses in the way that suits them best[2].

The policy of the SBC then is clear: fuel costs should normally be met from the scale rates. However, the SBC has always been loath to say what it considers a normal amount of expenditure on heating (or indeed any other commodity) to be:—

It is not possible to say how much of the scale rates is appropriate to any one item since this will depend both on the circumstances of the person, e.g. a young person may need to spend more on food and an older person more on fuel, and on his personal preferences...[3].

However, in practice, the SBC has found it necessary to have some figure in mind for heating costs. As the 1975 Annual Report explains:—

... in assessing benefit it has been necessary for the Commission for certain purposes to assume fixed amounts for heating or for all fuel costs, for example, in calculating a net rent where the rent paid is inclusive of heating...

... These sums are not − as they are sometimes described − the amounts included in the scale rates for heating and fuel. The level of the scale rates varies with family size. The overall amounts available for expenditure on heating and other commodities will vary accordingly and, as there is a significant element of personal choice in the level of heating it is ultimately a matter for the individual claimant what proportion of his income is allocated to heating.[4]

Weekly additions

Weekly 'discretionary additions' were a feature of means-tested assistance prior to the introduction of supplementary benefits following the 1966 Social Security Act. Indeed in the days of the National Assistance Board very large numbers of such additions were paid out.

In 1965 − the last full year of the National Assistance Board − over £30 million was spent giving 2,210,000 discretionary additions to 1,157,000 recipients − 58% of all national assistance cases (i.e. both pensioners and non-pensioners). Of this total 640,000 additions were for special diet, 520,000 for laundry, 268,000 for domestic help and 669,000 for extra fuel.[5]

The framers of the 1966 legislation thought this degree of discretion was doubly undesirable: large numbers of claimants should not have to rely on extra discretionary additions to make ends meet every week; and it was administratively time-consuming. A 'long-term addition' was consequently introduced in order to meet the needs of most, the intention being to restrict the additions to only a small minority − i.e. those with 'exceptional circumstances'.

The long-term addition

The purpose of the long-term addition is to provide a margin, over and above the ordinary level of requirements, for extra expenses of the kind which may be expected to arise in the generality of long-term cases. This addition is helpful both to the claimant and the Commission because it diminishes the need to make specific detailed enquiries about what can be quite small items of expense.[6]

The long-term addition (LTA) was awarded to virtually all supplementary pensioners and to other 'long-term' recipients of supplementary benefits. At the time of the 1972 Survey pensioners received an extra 60p a week, 85p where the claimant or a dependent was aged 80 or over.

An understanding of the reasons for introducing the LTA is important when we later consider the controversy over the relationship between the award of an ECA and the LTA. At this stage we need to note that the introduction of the LTA was effective in reducing the number of extra additions awarded. Thus in 1968 there were some 527,000 supplementary benefit cases with ECAs compared to 2,210,000 additions awarded in 1965 under national assistance.

Fuel allowances

While studies have been made into the financial circumstances of old people in general[7] and supplementary pensioners in particular,[8] there has been less interest, until recently, in the granting of exceptional circumstances additions: one of the most discretionary areas of social policy.

Before discussing the social circumstances that warrant the granting of an extra fuel addition it is necessary to look at the relationship between this addition and the main amount paid out as supplementary benefit. This relationship has changed since our survey in 1972.

Prior to the passing of the 1973 National Insurance and Supplementary Benefits Act, the LTA was taken into account in the operation of ECAs. As the handbook explained:—

> The special expenses of the beneficiary and his dependents are added up. Where the long-term addition applies, 50p (where the long-term addition is 60p), or 75p (where it is 85p) is deducted. The discretionary addition will then equal the remainder.[9]

And this, of course, could well be nothing: for example, a pensioner eligible for an ECA of 30p would get no extra money after account was taken of 50p of the LTA. In fact the 'eligible' pensioner would benefit financially only if he or she was awarded an ECA at the higher levels or if ECAs were awarded for more than one item.

The administrative logic behind these calculations is clear. The 1966 Social Security Act introduced the LTA to meet many of the extra expenses that were formerly covered by ECAs. It was therefore logical to take LTAs into account. But while the logic is incontestable the effects of the policy were controversial. Criticism was made on different grounds. One was that the procedure was misunderstood by elderly claimants. Few of these would have appreciated the idealistic origins of the LTA and its purpose.[10] Tony Lynes has given a good example of what could happen. A pensioner needed an extra 75p for heating and laundry. As this was more than 50p, a discretionary addition of 25p was awarded to cover the difference. But on reaching the age of 80 the pensioner would get the higher LTA (an extra 25p) while losing the 25p ECA since the whole cost of his extra needs was now covered by the LTA. As Lynes comments: 'It is all perfectly logical, but not very easy to explain.'[11]

The procedure was also attacked on the basis that at this low level of income every penny counts and, hence, every extra penny is welcome. The 'now you see it, now you don't' policy of 'awarding' an ECA (actually, recognizing a 'reckonable expense') and then offsetting it against the LTA is inhumane, it was argued, in this context. The procedure may be administratively correct and even 'right' in principle, but explaining that to an old lady denied her extra 30p would prove a difficult job: she may consider it downright mean.

The Simper case

The debate about the relationship between the LTA and ECAs came to focus around the interpretation of one phrase in the 1966 Ministry of Social Security Act. In schedule 2 of the Act, paragraph 4 (2) (a) states:

> In determining whether to award benefit in accordance with sub-para. (i) (a) [i.e. ECAs] regard shall be had to the provisions made by this schedule for additional requirements. [the LTA]

As has been said, the SBC interpreted this as meaning that one award must be deducted from the other. However critics argued that the legalistic phraseology did not have this precise meaning, but merely that some account had to be taken of the LTA.

In February 1973 the dispute was taken to the Queen's Bench Division of the High Court.[12] Mrs Simper, who had one child, had been receiving benefit since 1969 and was soon awarded an extra 35p a week for heating. After two years she qualified for an LTA of 50p a week, but in fact received only 15p more. A supplementary benefits appeals tribunal decided that her supplementary allowance had been properly calculated. She appealed against this decision to the High Court. Her counsel argued that the

Commission had laid down a hard and fast rule that where two additional sums were involved, as in the present case, there must always be a deduction from one. He submitted however that the correct interpretation of the paragraphs was that the assessing officer had a discretion. It did not mean that there had always to be an arithmetical deduction. Counsel acting on behalf of the Department of Health and Social Security argued that the paragraph was mandatory in the sense, not only that attention must be paid to the other sum, but also that a deduction must be made.

In giving his decision Mr Justice Cusack took the view that the paragraph meant that a discretion was to be exercised – that the person determining the sum to be paid should exercise his broad judgment to ensure that there was no overlap of payments. He ought not to proceed on a rule of thumb that a deduction must be made. Mr Justice Croom-Johnson and the Lord Chief Justice agreed. This legal victory was a great fillip to organizations such as the Child Poverty Action Group whose Citizens' Rights Office had taken up this case. The Heating Action Group, formed in 1972, was at this time organizing a campaign to put a large number of appeals before tribunals.[13]

Reform

Following the Simper case the Government was anxious generally to restore the position whereby ECAs are offset against most of the extra weekly amounts paid to 'long-term' claimants. The National Insurance and Supplementary Benefits Bill was changed to achieve this. However, three exceptions were made, one being heating additions.[14] In future long-term claimants were to receive the full amount of any ECA for heating. This welcome, though anomalous, decision was no doubt due to a reluctance to overturn directly the High Court's ruling and a concern to give some extra help with heating costs in the wake of growing anxiety about the 'hypothermia' issue. A major effect of this change of policy was a great increase in the number of ECAs paid for extra heating.

The National Insurance and Supplementary Benefits Act 1973 also introduced 'long-term weekly rates' in place of the scale rates plus LTA that applied previously. Thus at November 1976 a single pensioner claimant aged under 80 received £15.70 and one aged 80 or over £15.95 (compared to £12.70 for a younger person on the 'ordinary weekly rate').

Exceptional circumstances

The awarding of weekly additions for heating has been subject to a number of changes over the years. These changes relate to the seasonal times of payment; the amount of the addition; and the criteria for the award.

For most of its life the National Assistance Board only awarded fuel additions during the winter months. This policy was based on the argument that the scale rates included provision for 'average normal heating requirements throughout the whole year' according to the Board's Report for 1965. Nevertheless some people had:—

> ... a special need of heating during the winter months, e.g. because of ill-health or damp or draughty accommodation, and it has for many years been the practice to make an addition to their allowances for this purpose from November to April inclusive.[15]

Nevertheless, following representations from organizations representing old people, the Board decided that in future there would be a uniform addition (at half the winter rate) throughout the year. This practice has also been followed under supplementary benefits.

Another change of practice has involved the basis for assessing the amount of the addition. Under national assistance, and from 1966 to 1970 for supplementary benefits, fuel allowances were based on the price of coal. There were two rates, the equivalent of either a quarter or a half of a hundredweight of coal (at local prices). In 1970 the SBC reviewed their policy on heating additions and three rates for heating additions (or, more correctly, standard amounts of reckonable expenses) were introduced. The amounts were one quarter, one half and three-quarters (at that time, 25p, 50p and 75p) of what 'it would be reasonable to expect a person living on supplementary benefit to spend on heating' (i.e. the assumed amount referred to earlier).[16] Since their introduction these amounts have been uprated in line with movements of the fuel component in the Retail Prices Index.

A third area that has been the subject of change concerns the criteria for awarding heating additions. The major grounds for an award have traditionally concerned the ill-health or immobility of the claimant and the difficulty of keeping accommodation warm. The criteria were extended in 1970 and, since then, have been spelt out in greater detail (see below).

A more contemporary issue relates to the changing patterns of heating. Coal is the traditional fuel and has always been of particular importance for the poor. The practice of basing heating addition figures on coal prices reflects this. But the advent of central heating, brought to the poor with new local authority housing, has posed new problems. As we have seen, heating additions have usually been awarded on the basis of exceptional need (i.e. poor health or housing that is difficult to heat) rather than cost of fuel itself (although need and cost will obviously be related). Costs and the existence of fixed charges have necessitated a different approach towards claimants with central heating.

Until 1975 it was the practice to award ECAs where a claimant's central heating costs exceeded a standard figure:—

> An extra heating addition will be made if, on the basis of guidance from local fuel authorities, or by reference to any fixed regular charges that are made, the necessary expenditure on central heating can be expected to exceed that figure.

This policy was reviewed in 1975 and revised because, according to the SBC:—

> It had been complicated to administer and to keep up to date, and it had provided no additional help to any older person inclined to economise in the use of central heating.[17]

In practice however, worries about the open-ended nature of the provision and its abuse (central heating full on, open windows) were additional powerful arguments in favour of reform. It was therefore decided to introduce standard additions according to the size of the centrally heated dwelling. When a fixed charge is payable, however, the amount of an ECA is the difference between this and the SBC's assumed amount for heating.

The DHSS leaflet *'Help with Heating Costs'* (November 1976) details the formula governing the award of heating additions and it is worth reproducing it in full:—

> The following extra heating additions are payable for you or a dependant where:
>
> (1) mobility is restricted because of general frailty or advanced age   70p
> (2) extra heating is required because of chronic ill-health (e.g. chronic bronchitis, rheumatism, severe anaemia or chronic debility)   70p
> (3) one of you is housebound (or mobility is so restricted that one of you is unable to leave the house unaided)   £1.40
> (4) there is serious illness requiring extra heating   £1.40
> (5) one of you is bedfast (or mobility is so restricted that assistance in walking in the room is required) and extra heating is needed day and night   £2.10
> (6) because of serious illness a constant room temperature is required day and night   £2.10

or if you are a householder and:

(7)   the accommodation is difficult to heat adequately (e.g.
       on account of damp or because the rooms are unusually
       large)   70p

(8)   the nature and condition of the accommodation is such
       that it is exceptionally difficult to heat adequately   £1.40

Any one of the amounts numbered (1−6) may be added to either one of the
amounts numbered (7 and 8) subject to an overall maximum addition of £2.10. In
very exceptional cases an addition of more than £2.10 may be made.

CENTRAL HEATING

If you are occupying centrally heated accommodation an extra heating addition
will be made, normally according to the number of rooms (bedrooms, living-
rooms and kitchen) as follows:—

       1 or 2 rooms   35p
       3 or 4 rooms   70p
       5 or more rooms   £1.40

If you pay a fixed charge for central heating any addition payable will depend on
the amount of the charge.

Numbers

We have discussed a number of shifts in official policy towards the award
of heating additions in recent years. These changes have had an important
impact on their scope. The total number of cases with a heating ECA has
increased from 194,000 in 1971 to 1,100,000 in May 1976 and for supplementary pensioners the respective figures are 159,000 and 912,000. The
last figures represent an increase from 8% to 55% of all supplementary
pensioners.[18] There has been a general increase in all ECAs during this
period, but their growing importance is fundamentally due to the increase
in heating addition awards.

Some of the immediate causes of the increase have been considered.
The change in the relationship between heating ECAs and the LTA was a
major factor and it was due to outside pressure, culminating in the Simper
case, that the DHSS reluctantly gave in. Another important factor, reflecting public opinion, has been a more sympathetic approach by the SBC. A
reluctance to award fuel allowances − treating them as truly *exceptional*
circumstances additions − has made way for a more generous strategy
whereby it is probable that an old person applying for an ECA is more,
rather than less, likely to receive one. Today over half of all supplementary pensioners receive heating additions, the vast majority of
them on health grounds. Given greater publicity and more applications

this proportion would be significantly higher. In fact the SBC's Inspectorate undertook a survey in the winter of 1975/76 that found that while 49% of supplementary pensioners were receiving heating additions, as many as 75% appeared to have satisfied the criteria for receiving one. This means that, at the beginning of 1975, there may have been 400,000 pensioners not receiving the help they should have got.[19] But if ECAs are no longer 'exceptional', and if there is now a major exercise of discretion in this area of supplementary benefits, is this good news or bad news? The implications of this development for the old and cold problem are considered in the conclusion to this chapter. However it is useful to discuss first its importance for the supplementary benefits system as a whole.

Discretion

The SBC is, in part, a 'safety-net' agency and, arguably, as such it must be able to exercise discretion. For instance certain individual needs, a special diet for example, will have to be paid for – hence ECAs.

In the case of heating additions the supplementary benefits officer is guided by both general policy and numerous instructions. The general criteria (listed above) for awarding ECAs for heating are both detailed and complex (and certainly difficult for the ordinary claimant to understand). There are also detailed instructions set out in the 'A' Code (frequently up-dated and changed) that officers have to follow.

Nevertheless this still leaves a good deal of 'officer discretion'.[20] For example, what does 'adequately' heated mean? Would this include the bedroom? Would a room temperature of below 70°F be considered 'inadequate'? (as one DHSS leaflet would imply).[21] Another example is mobility. What does 'restricted' mean here? To raise such questions is not to imply that greater clarity, and hence standardization in administration, would be easy, for discretion, by its very nature, makes this difficult. But such questions do show the problems that face benefits officers and the barriers preventing claimants from fully comprehending the system. Is this heavy reliance on discretion satisfactory?

The SBC's Chairman, David Donnison, has argued that the country has to choose:—

> It can either go for more discretion, more flexibility, a labour-intensive service and 'creative justice' for individual claimants, or it can go for more uniformity, more clearly understood civil rights, fewer civil servants, and 'proportional justice' for large categories of claimants. We cannot have both and to try for both ... leads only to chaos and recrimination.[22].

In order to be able to judge what choice should be made, it is useful to discuss the advantages and disadvantages of discretion in terms of flexibility; knowledge; complexity and ignorance; 'rights'; equity; and administration and costs.

Flexibility

As argued above the idea of a 'safety net' agency implies a certain level of discretion in the award of cash allowances. While the legislation of 1966 was largely based on a concept of 'entitlement', emphasizing the rights of claimants, discretionary weekly additions were nevertheless retained and, in practice, the argument is more about their scope than about their existence. Probably the major advantage of discretion is its flexibility. Richard Titmuss has argued that the additional grants under supplementary benefits 'allow flexible responses to human needs and to an immense variety of complex individual circumstances'.[23] A scheme without discretion would not allow for 'individual justice' because 'a definition of entitlement in precise material and itemised terms would deprive the recipient of choice, and by prohibiting flexibility would mean that whatever the level of provision it would become maximum which no official or tribunal could exceed.'[24]

Olive Stevenson has also argued the case for some discretion in terms of 'creative' justice which is 'concerned with the uniqueness and therefore the differential need of individuals'.[25] However, there is a danger of exaggerating the degree of flexibility allowed, in practice, by the supplementary benefits system. Few claimants would probably recognize in its exercise of discretion the practical implementation of 'individualized' or 'creative' justice. More modestly ECAs can be said to bring about a certain flexibility in relation to certain needs and hence recognize the variability of individual circumstances.

Knowledge

A less obvious, but important, spin-off from the exercise of discretion is the knowledge or feed-back gained by the SBC and officers. By getting involved in difficult problems such as heating, the needs for special diets, clothing requirements and so on, government officials come face to face every day with the reality of contemporary poverty. The knowledge so gained can complement more scientific sources such as Family Expenditure Survey data and survey findings in helping the DHSS and SBC understand financial hardship and the appropriate balance between entitlement and discretion. Discussions within government in recent years have been, arguably, better informed and certainly more urgent because of the supplementary benefits system's continuing task of dealing with such issues as inadequate heating and disconnections. Knowledge gained through discretion can lead to innovation and its potential here has been discussed by both Titmuss and Bull.[26] The introduction of the LTA in 1966 is one example.

Complexity and ignorance

Discretion, then, does have advantages. But what are the possible disadvantages? One of the most obvious is the complexity discretion can bring to a system of cash assistance. Although a discretionary system is not necessarily a complex one (and other systems are certainly not necessarily free of complexity) in practice discretion tends to complexity and this is certainly the case with supplementary benefits (as its secret codes testify).

Complexity often means that claimants are ignorant about the actual workings of discretion. Furthermore, there may be ignorance about the very existence of discretionary powers. Our own survey revealed that 74% of supplementary pensioners not claiming to receive additions did not know they existed and this ignorance is confirmed by the finding that only 3% reported receiving such ECAs (when many more were almost certainly receiving them). These results are hardly surprising when a quarter of those eligible fail to claim supplementary pensions. But ignorance is only the first barrier. Who can claim? How to claim? When to claim? What (exactly) to claim? It is uncertainty about the answers to such questions – and sometimes even an inability to formulate the questions – that prevents some claimants from understanding and making use of discretionary procedures. Nor should it be assumed that the present system is easy for social security staff to understand. In fact many staff consider the instructions about heating additions to be very complex and sometimes hard to interpret.

Given the present system of ECAs for heating, the task of explaining the system is not an easy one, although there is a role for the right kind of publicity and welfare rights campaign (as discussed later). Its likely impact is, however, unlikely to be substantial.

Rights?

How does discretion affect the concept of entitlement? The intention of the 1966 Act was that claimants should have a positive right to benefits. As we have seen, discretion would affect a small minority. But the growth of ECAs over recent years represents a significant change.

Richard Titmuss has stated that one of the general principles relevant to the Commission's attempts to find a balance 'between precision and flexibility, rule and discretion' is that 'people should be helped to know their rights.'[27] The relationship between discretion and rights, between flexibility and entitlement is a difficult and complex one.

But do discretionary additions increase rights? It is difficult to be convinced. We have seen that there is a good deal of ignorance about ECAs for heating. Given this, can we speak of a right to an ECA? And is it just ignorance or complexity that prevents claims? Some clients are unwilling to apply. Perhaps originally uncertain or unhappy about applying for supplementary benefit itself, many (supplementary) pensioners are loath to ask for help. Pride, independence or a worry about what friends and neighbours would think (should they hear) can all combine to prevent a claim. All of these factors were relevant to one old lady whom the author met. In addition she had not heard of heating additions and certainly would not have known how to apply for one. And while her home was cold and fuel bills a worry, this lady also half-felt that 'things were not too bad' and she was full of gratitude for the supplementary pension she did get. Only strong persuasion and a letter written on her behalf led to a claim being made (which was promptly and positively responded to).

Much can be done (and has been done) to make claiming and the handling of a claim relatively simple and trouble-free. But any system of this kind involves the asking of questions (which most citizens are not called upon to answer) and is bound to invade privacy. Can we be proud of a system where people have to ask for extra money to buy essentials, be they blankets, shoes for children or extra warmth? Are not such requests – and the institutions, policies and procedures thrown up for dealing with them – likely further to isolate the poor from the rest of the population and to divide rather than unite society?

Equity

The exercise of discretion inevitably leads to inconsistency of administration: this means the unfair or inequitable treatment of one citizen compared to the next. This basic problem pre-dates the SBC. Michael Hill has noted that:—

> The National Assistance Board was required to maintain people at a low subsistence level. At that level people differ markedly from each other in their basic needs. The Board was required to take into account these differences and thus it had to give discretionary powers to those of its officers who were actually meeting the public. Thus it was inevitable that in a relationship in which individual officers were required to size up the needs of individual applicants for help one would find inconsistency.[28]

What was true for the NAB is also true for the SBC. That inconsistency is 'inevitable' is hardly surprising when one looks at the problems involved. It is worth noting Hill's comments on fuel allowances. After discussing consistency when it came to laundry expenses and the 'even more haphazard' special diet allowances, Hill states:

> The amounts of fuel allowances . . . were standardised by managerial edict; the difficulty here was to achieve any consistency about who should have them. Officers were required to take into account the general health and mobility of the applicant, together with the state of his or her accommodation. Naturally, it was impossible for any clear rules to be laid down on the evaluation of factors of this kind.[29]

It would seem likely that a substantial proportion of supplementary beneficiaries who do receive heating additions are in fact receiving them at the wrong level. One can then talk about the exercise of discretion in terms of its implication for equity and fairness. But to point to inevitable *inequities* and *unfairness* is, perhaps, to give only half the argument. The SBC's Annual Report for 1975 has noted that 'with the best of intentions, the Commission and the government have tended to assume that every exceptional case should ideally be dealt with in a uniform way in every part of the country: it is regarded almost as a scandal if anyone can show that he or those whom he represents are treated less generously than other people with similar needs.'[30] But to guard against this leads inevitably to rules, regulations and complexity. The Commission notes that 'where discretion remains we must consider whether we should tolerate more variety in the ways in which it is interpreted and give greater autonomy to local offices which would no longer be expected to treat every type of exception in uniform ways.'[31]

Administration and costs

One specific disadvantage of more and more ECAs has been noted by the SBC:—

> Discretion, because it makes decisions harder, and calls for experienced officials and a lot of visiting, is very expensive in staff to administer properly.[32]

At any time administration and cost factors will be important in the debate about discretion. The current pressure to reduce public expenditure and, consequently, the number of civil servants, allied to extremely difficult social security staff problems, can only increase their significance. Referring to discretionary additions, David Donnison has warned that: 'The whole tottering Christmas tree threatens to collapse under its own weight.'[33]

Policy Alternatives

Many elderly people do not have enough money to spend on heating and a large number of these are supplementary pensioners. The current system of ECAs for fuel is, however, an ineffective and undesirable way of meeting the problem. On the assumption therefore that reform is required, what policy alternatives exist? The options range from the piecemeal and relatively cheap to the grand and expensive and not all are mutually exclusive.

Reformed ECAs

The first possibility to consider is the reform of the ECA system. Any such reform should aim, firstly, to make heating additions more intelligible to the claimant and, secondly, to increase awareness of the benefit and hence take-up rates. The major advantage of this option is that it offers a means of selectively aiding many of the elderly who are most in need. Furthermore, this selective assistance could be given relatively inexpensively.

The reform embodied in the 1973 National Insurance and Supplementary Benefit Act whereby extra heating additions are *not* offset against the new scale rates for long-term claimants certainly makes the system more intelligible. One source of confusion (and exasperation) has been removed.

What further initiatives are necessary? One might be the greater systematization of eligibility. But one must recognize straightaway that this, by definition, erodes discretion and therefore reduces flexibility. In his critique of the increasing application of 'legality' to the public assistance system in the United States, Titmuss has stated that:—

> Itemised legal entitlements, in the assessment of needs and resources, now embrace hundreds of visible articles and objects − practically everything that bedrooms, living-rooms, kitchens and lavatories may contain.[34]

Whether or not such developments are desirable it is easier to be specific about such things as household commodities and clothing than about heating and warmth. Nor would greater systematization necessarily make for greater clarity. It would no doubt be possible to make instructions to supplementary benefits officers even more specific and to publish these. But while such specificity would help the lay representative it might further complicate the system for the claimant himself and lead to more confusion – how many claimants can now fully understand the (rather detailed) eligibility criteria laid down? It would also make the system more complicated for staff to administer and might increase staff numbers, at a time when all the pressure is on the need to reduce staff.

Notwithstanding these problems, the criteria for the granting of extra fuel additions could be positively changed. Target groups might be identified such as the very aged – the over 80s, say.[35] Everyone in these groups could be awarded an ECA (i.e. a move from discretion to entitlement). Alternatively, persons in the groups could have their circumstances specially reviewed to see whether eligibility for an ECA existed. This would certainly involve staff in more contact with supplementary pensioners. The reduction in home visiting by supplementary benefits officers in recent years has inevitably meant that many cases of need go undetected and therefore unmet. Postal reviews, while relatively inexpensive, can be less efficient than face-to-face contact. Following a change in criteria of eligibility, case papers are not always scrutinised to see if an award should now be made, nor does sufficient information always exist on file to allow a decision to be taken.

Greater publicity for the ECA system is essential. Advertising should include not only the provision of leaflets, posters and so on – although these are very important – but also special briefings for supplementary benefits officers, social workers, housing managers and staff of both statutory and voluntary bodies. Efforts have been made in recent years to publicise ECAs for fuel. Part of the criteria laid down in the 'A' code has, since 1972, been published in the *Supplementary Benefits Handbook*. Also a special leaflet 'Help with Heating Costs' has been published by the Department of Health and Social Security.

The Supplementary Benefits Commission reviewed publicity again in 1976, and, in the light of their Inspectorate's survey findings (referred to earlier), took three steps to increase public awareness. First, local office staff were asked to give special attention to the possible need of those without heating additions. Second, a poster was issued for display in post offices and doctors' waiting rooms. And third, the DHSS Regional Information Officers were asked to take measures to increase public knowledge of heating additions.[36]

Given the scale and severity of the problems faced by the elderly and cold, publicity in the past has been frankly half-hearted and lacking in urgency. Television could play an important role and there is a need for advertising on this medium, at least on a trial-run basis. Television and certain other forms of advertising can create problems – the raising of false hopes, claimants that have to be disappointed and pressure on local offices. But these are justified if a significant number of extra awards to those most in need do result from the publicity.

Exceptional needs payments

This chapter has concentrated on ECAs. It is important briefly to discuss, however, the potential of the other form of discretionary award – the exceptional needs payment. Whereas ECAs provide help with weekly heating costs, the award of an ENP might tackle the problem at its root, by enabling more efficient heating appliances to be purchased, for example.

ENPs are lump-sum payments to claimants, made only occasionally. During 1976 288,000 ENPs were awarded to supplementary pensioners, the average amount being £18.89.[37] These payments are based on the recognition that claimants, particularly those reliant on benefit for a long period of time, will occasionally need to renew certain household goods. ENPs are awarded as it is realized that such expenses could not be met from the weekly allowance. ENPs are most commonly awarded to meet the cost of such items as clothing and footwear, bedding, and removal expenses. They are referred to in the DHSS leaflet 'Help with Heating Costs' which states that:—

> Sometimes the need for extra warmth can be met by, for example, extra blankets, repair or replacement of an ineffective heating appliance, or materials for draught-proofing (where a relative, friend, or voluntary worker can do the necessary work if you are unable to do so). In this case you may be able to get a single discretionary lump-sum payment if you have £200 or less in savings.

Heating equipment is not separately listed in the SBC's 1973 report on ENPs[38] and one suspects that little use has been made of ENPs for such a purpose. It is hoped that the SBC will in future encourage the greater use of ENPs for more 'preventive' help than is possible through the granting of ECAs.

The implications of this, however, have to be seen in terms of the powers and responsibilities of other agencies and these are discussed in our concluding chapter. We will also consider there the policy implications of our findings (see Chapter 5) that electric blankets seem, on the available evidence, to be a relatively effective measure in the fight against hypothermia.

Recipients of supplementary benefit (including non-pensioners) at the end of 1975 had received in the previous 12 months 42,000 ENPs for fuel, the average payment being £22.70.[39] The SBC are extremely reluctant to meet fuel bills and where they do the circumstances are looked at very carefully and steps taken in the hope that the situation will not arise again. The fact, however, that fuel bills are occasionally met by the SBC would seem to underline the case for a more positive approach to the whole question of heating costs and heating standards. This argument is pursued in Chapter 9 where the SBC's current approach to the problem of fuel debts is also noted.

Paying full heating costs

An increasing expansion of discretionary heating additions is not the best way of meeting the heating needs of the cold elderly. In any case the signs strongly suggest that in future we will see less discretion in supplementary benefits, rather than more. The 1976 Annual Report deplores the trends towards discretion and argues that it erodes confidence:—

> the confidence of claimants that they have clearly defined rights to benefit, the confidence of staff that they are getting extra money to those who really need it most, and the confidence of the public that we are being fair to claimants and non-claimants alike.[40]

The major disadvantage of discretionary heating additions is that many eligible claimants do not receive them. Even the most imaginative promotional policy would probably fail to tackle this problem adequately. A more direct approach to the meeting of heating costs is therefore worth discussing.

Supplementary benefit consists in part of a payment for housing costs. In most cases a claimant's full housing costs are taken into account when assessing benefit entitlement. Might not heating be treated in a similar way? The special treatment of housing is due to the fact that the cost of it can vary tremendously from one household to the next through no fault of the individuals concerned. For example, two supplementary pensioners may live in identical houses. One has lived there since before the war and pays a controlled rent of only 75p a week; the other moved in during the 1960s and pays a rent of £5 a week. Justifiably the State meets the full housing costs of both in order that a high rent does not completely distort the weekly budgets of old people. Similarly it could be argued that heating costs often vary from case to case through no fault of the individuals concerned, due to house type, heating equipment, bad insulation, etc. Given such variation there would seem to be a case for the State meeting the heating costs of supplementary benefit recipients. The high costs of heating, and not just the variation in costs, would support such a policy.

This approach would prevent an old person with high heating bills from going without adequate heating or else perhaps cutting down expenditure on other necessities such as food. There might well be a legitimate argument against paying the full heating costs on the grounds that the scale rates already include a heating element. In this case the policy could be to pay heating costs over and above this amount which is already allowed for. This is still the approach adopted towards many of those with central heating.

There is no doubt that such a policy would be very much harder to administer than the similar one for housing. Heating costs would in some cases be harder for the claimant to calculate and for the Commission to verify. Nevertheless, in principle, this would seem to be a logical and humane approach to the problem and for these reasons deserves further consideration.

Higher scale rates

An alternative to the reform of weekly fuel allowances is to increase supplementary benefits scale rates to such an extent that extra fuel additions – and ECAs generally for that matter – could be abolished. The advantages of this strategy relate to coverage and administration. The need to prove entitlement to extra help with fuel costs would vanish and everyone on supplementary benefit would in principle be adequately protected. It would also reduce the administrative load on supplementary benefits officers – no insignificant advantage – and base the system more on 'rights' than discretion.

The approach is open to a number of objections however. Firstly, cost. It would be very much more expensive than a reform of ECAs for a number of reasons. The costs would include the extra benefits for existing claimants; the cost of benefits to the newly eligible (as a result of raising levels); or the cost of corresponding national insurance pension increases (required to prevent the increase in social security rolls). Even a limited increase in scale rates would be very expensive. The SBC has calculated that to give all supplementary pensioners an increase in their weekly benefit equivalent to the average value of ECAs now paid to over half of them would cost £40 million a year.[41] A second disadvantage of this approach is that it would probably fail to offer enough help to those elderly persons at present receiving relatively large ECAs for central heating. Thirdly, it is a strategy based on supplementary benefits and is (together with the other policy options so far discussed) consequently open to fundamental objections.

A means-tested solution?

Improvements to the system of heating additions, the payment of 'full' heating costs or an improvement in scale rates would all offer some help to present and future claimants of supplementary benefit. Nevertheless a fundamental objection to such options is that they could do nothing for the estimated 600,000 pensioners who (in December 1975) appeared to be eligible for supplementary benefit but were not receiving it.[42] For this reason none of the policy options so far mentioned would seem desirable, seeking as they do to find a solution to heating problems within the context of the means-test. Titmuss has stated that one of the principles of a more humane supplementary benefits system is the need to reduce the scope and coverage: 'already it has too many claimants, too many callers, too many clients, too large a case-load.'[43]

Another fundamental problem concerns equity. The supplementary benefit standard offers, at best, a crude and unscientific dividing line between one group of citizens and the next. Pensioners just above this line are not well-off. As our survey shows, many of the old not receiving benefit have low body temperatures and/or suffer from cold conditions. 'Solutions' to the problem of the cold need to be found for all those in need (whatever their social security status) and this calls for a more universal approach.

Higher pensions

By far the most attractive policy option is a substantial increase in pensions. The inadequacy of existing pensions is the major cause of poverty in old age and the reason for the dependency of so many old people on supplementary benefits. Although subject to periodic increases the pension as a proportion of net average earnings has remained broadly the same since the mid-1960s, although there has been an improvement in recent years.[44]

Several policies have been proposed which would result in a reduction in the numbers dependent on means-testing. For example, one of the effects of the Tax-Credit scheme was officially reckoned to be that 'something like a million national insurance beneficiaries, most of them retirement pensioners, might have their incomes raised above supplementary benefit levels. This would reduce the numbers drawing a supplementary pension by over a third.'[45] More directly the pension plans of both Conservative and Labour Administrations would reduce means-testing in old age. The proposals set out in the White Paper 'Better Pensions',[46] now enacted in the Social Security Pensions Act 1975 will, in time, achieve this objective. But in time! Whatever the advantages (or disadvantages) of the different pension schemes of the last decade they have nothing to offer today's pensioner.

To complement this long-term social planning, there is an urgent need to help existing pensioners and to meet directly the contemporary poverty of the old. A substantial increase in basic pensions is the only solution. Pension increases are usually accompanied by similar increases in supplementary benefit rates and consequently the approximate number of elderly claiming benefits remains the same. Herein lies a major dilemma: if pension rates are raised, but supplementary benefit levels are not, two things will happen: (i) the numbers on benefit will decrease and (ii) many of the poorest pensioners (those remaining on benefit) will not gain from the pension increase. A way of making this dilemma less painful is to phase out dependency on supplementary benefits gradually. Each time basic pensions are increased, supplementary benefits could be too, but by a lesser amount. Over, say, a five-year period means-testing in old age could be abolished. The main beneficiaries of this strategy will be the group containing the poorer elderly: those eligible for supplementary benefit, but not claiming it.

How much would a policy such as this cost? Some indication can be given. It was officially estimated (in 1974) that the raising of national insurance pensions by £2 for a single person and £2.75 for a married couple would take 750,000 retirement pensioners off supplementary benefit at a net cost of £565 million a year.[47]

The strategy advocated here would be enormously expensive. The cost could only be met by the redistribution of substantial resources from rich to poor and from young to old. Ultimately, however, this is the only sure way of mounting an effective attack on poverty in old age, which is so closely related to the problem of the 'old and cold'.

Policy

Chapter 8
Personal Social Services
(with Anthony Hall)*

Much of this book has been concerned with analysing the medical and social problem of hypothermia, and identifying the conditions and circumstances under which the old and cold live. Any effective policy to combat these problems will obviously involve the work of and co-operation between a number of agencies, both statutory and voluntary, at central and local levels. The local authority social services department, however, has an essential and special role to play. It has the primary responsibility for defining needs in the community, and for protecting 'at risk' groups; it is also arguably in the best position to co-ordinate services, promote the expansion of facilities and ensure the full utilization of the benefits available.

This chapter explores the current and potential roles of social services departments in dealing with the problems of the cold elderly. It draws upon the findings of a small study of the policies and practices of London boroughs conducted by the two authors of this chapter in the summer of 1974. In particular our enquiries focused upon three main issues:

1. What are local authority social services departments able to do under existing legislation?
2. What kind of central direction, help or encouragement have they received? And, against this background,
3. What are social services departments actually doing for the cold elderly?

Legislation

What are local authority social services departments able to do for the cold elderly, given the existing legislation? The answer to this first question is fairly straightforward. Under existing legislation social services departments can do almost anything to relieve the plight of this group. The levels of provision and the rate of service development have far more to do with competition in priorities with other need groups than with legislative

*Lecturer in Social Administration, University of Bristol.

119

constraints. This has not always been the case, but the powers of local welfare authorities in relation to the needs of the elderly have been extended considerably since the war, and over the last 15 years in particular.

For much of the post-war period the care of the elderly was primarily determined by two pieces of legislation: the National Assistance Act, 1948 and the National Health Service Act, 1946. Both statutes contained major reforms: the former, the abolition of the poor law and the establishment of the National Assistance Board with responsibility for financially assisting those in need; the latter, the introduction of the tripartite National Health Service. In both measures the welfare provisions for the elderly took a back seat, and this reflects the general lack of coherence in planning for their care. Despite the stirring statement of the 1948 Act that from the appointed day 'The existing poor law shall cease to have effect', the early post-war reforms made little impact on social welfare provisions for the old. They meant little more than a reordering of organizational boundaries and responsibilities for existing services.

Under the National Assistance Act, 1948, county and county borough councils were given two duties. First, they had a responsibility to provide residential accommodation 'for persons who by reasons of age, infirmity or any other circumstances are in need of care or attention which is not otherwise available to them': second they were to provide temporary accommodation for anyone needing it 'in circumstances which could not reasonably have been foreseen or in such other circumstances as the local authority may in any particular case determine'.[1]

No provision was made in the Act directly promoting or facilitating domiciliary services for the care of the elderly, but Part III, section 29(1) states: 'A local authority shall have power to make arrangements for promoting the welfare of persons to whom this section applies, that is to say to persons who are blind, deaf or dumb and other persons who are substantially and permanently handicapped by illness, injury or congenital deformity or such other disabilities as may be prescribed by the Minister.' Although this provision did not specifically refer to the elderly, some of the elderly most at risk were covered by it.[2] Certain domiciliary provisions were made possible under the National Health Service Act, 1946, which amongst other things enabled local authority health departments to provide home help and nursing services, but with these few exceptions an authority could only provide domiciliary supports for the elderly indirectly by subsidies to local voluntary organizations. Indeed, only in 1962 under the National Assistance (Amendment) Act was a local authority able to provide recreational facilities and its own meals-on-wheels service.[3]

The post-war period has been characterized by an increasing emphasis on domiciliary care in principle, if not always in practice. This emphasis reflected in the health and welfare plans of the mid 1960s was eventually given a broad statutory base in the Health Services and Public Health Act, 1968. This Act gave a wide range of permissive powers to county, county borough and London borough councils and the equivalent local authorities in Scotland and Wales. One small part of this 'bits and pieces' measure gave these local authorities far more powers in relation to the elderly than the subsequent Seebohm legislation was able to provide for other need groups. Section 45(1) states: 'The local authority may with the approval of the Minister of Health and to such extent as he may direct, *make arrangements for promoting the welfare of old people*' (our italics).

By way of elaboration, during the second reading of the Bill, the Minister of Health, Kenneth Robinson, said that the powers envisaged included 'practical forms of help which can be given; houses can be adapted, and small personal services and aid offered, which will make it easier for elderly people to go on living in their own homes.' The new powers were intended to be 'as flexible as possible so that an authority will be free to develop its services as it wishes.' Unfortunately, despite these intentions, immediately after the Act was passed Circular 31/68 was issued announcing that the implementation of Section 45 would have to be delayed owing to the 'economic situation'. In the meantime authorities were urged:

> to review the welfare needs of elderly people in their areas; to form provisional views as to effective means, in collaboration with other statutory and voluntary services, of identifying those to whom services ought, in their view, primarily to be offered and as to the nature of those services; to consider how independent voluntary services can be assisted to expand and work in partnership with them in order to promote effective development.

To facilitate the development of this partnership, Section 65 of the Act extended the powers of local authorities to make grants or loans to voluntary organizations concerned with the care of the elderly, and to develop collaborative projects.

It was not until 1st April, 1971, that Section 45 of the 1968 Act came into force.[4] In a further Circular (19/71) issued by the Department of Health and Social Security it was said that 'the purpose of Section 45 is to enable authorities to make other approved arrangements of services to the elderly who are not substantially and permanently handicapped, and thus to promote the welfare of the elderly generally and as far as possible prevent or postpone personal deterioration or breakdown.'[5] It was not the Secretary of State's intention at this stage, however, to direct authorities to make arrangements. The circular stated that there were financial limitations on the use authorities would be able to make of their powers. Nevertheless, the Secretary of State approved of local authorities making arrangements for meeting the needs of the elderly under a variety of headings. These included the provision of meals and recreation in the home and elsewhere; information to the elderly about the services available; the provision of facilities or assistance for travelling in order to use available services; a boarding-out service; and the provision of visiting and advisory services and social work support. He was also prepared, as an interim measure, 'to consider proposals by individual authorities for the making of arrangements for services similar to the above, but his specific approval will be required for these.'[6]

In addition to these wide powers Circular 19/71 urged authorities 'to find out which of the elderly need help and what kind of help they need'[7] and, in providing services, to do so with 'the closest co-operation between those who are responsible for the various elements that make up the community health and social services.'[8] Given the limitations of resources, however, 'it may well prove desirable to start by identifying the needs of certain groups of the elderly who seem likely to be particularly vulnerable, e.g. (a) elderly people, especially the more elderly, who are housebound or living alone or recently bereaved or about to be discharged from hospital and (b) other persons over, say, 75 living in the community, particularly where there are high concentrations of very elderly people in particular districts.'[9]

The circular made no specific mention of the heating needs of the elderly, but local authorities were authorized 'to provide practical assistance in the carrying out of works of adaptation or *any additional facilities designed to secure greater safety, comfort or convenience*'[10] (our italics). Although this is a rather broad and vague statement, it could well be argued that the heating needs of the elderly are covered by it. A 'progressive' local authority, anxious and willing to provide, say, blankets, heating equipment or even insulation could point to this statement as giving them the power to do so.

The most recent legislative landmark was the 1970 Chronically Sick and Disabled Persons Act. This Act extends and strengthens immediate post-war legislation and requires local authorities 'to secure that they are adequately informed of the numbers and needs of substantially and permanently handicapped persons in order that they can formulate satisfactory plans for developing their services.'[11] They are also required to ensure that the handicapped are informed as to what help is available.[12] Again, some of these provisions could be seen as allowing local welfare authorities to provide help and aid with heating problems. In short, there are many opportunities for local authorities to develop a wide range of provisions to deal with the problems of the cold elderly. If by chance, or ministerial direction, a particular activity in relation to heating is deemed to be inappropriate or contrary to central policy, a concerned and determined local authority can still find a way of meeting needs as they see them. For example, as reported by Kathleen Slack, in 1972[13] a number of local authorities wished to use Section 45 of the 1968 Health Services and Public Health Act to pay the fuel bills of elderly persons in need, as is at present possible in Scotland. This request was refused by the Secretary of State for Social Services on the grounds that the Supplementary Benefits Commission already made adequate use of their powers to make discretionary payments in such cases. To avoid this limitation on the interpretation of the 1968 Act, one particularly determined London borough earmarked £500 of its grant to the Old People's Welfare Association for payments to any old person found to be in financial difficulty over heating costs.

Central Direction

What direction, encouragement or advice has central government provided to local authorities about the problem of the cold elderly? In August 1972 a joint circular from the Department of Health and Social Security and the Department of the Environment was issued: 'Heating for Elderly People in Winter'.[14] The circular began rather tentatively, and with at least one eye on the politics of welfare provision:

> Authorities will be aware of recent local surveys which have once again focused attention on the problems faced by some elderly people in keeping warm during the winter, and they will no doubt wish to consider what further action may be desirable and practicable in their areas to help in meeting these problems. The action required to meet all of them will clearly be long-term, and can only be taken to the extent that the many demands on manpower and other resources allow. In some cases, however, it may possible to make a beginning before next winter, and the purpose of this circular is to suggest some steps that might be taken and to offer such assistance as Departments can give in doing so.[15]

The circular warned that although all old people may be vulnerable to the cold, those at greatest risk appear to be 'those in the less active higher age groups (e.g. 75 or over) living alone – including elderly couples living alone – and particularly those who are housebound or severely handicapped.'[16] Authorities were encouraged to focus attention on this group, and voluntary organizations and local officers of the Supplementary Benefits Commission were seen as possible sources of information about those at risk. In addition it was suggested that they might take rather more direct action by contacting the local Executive Council 'who if approached at an early stage may be willing to assist by sending an explanatory letter prepared by the Social Services Authority to (say) all aged 75 or over on their list.'[17]

Whilst the emphasis of the circular was upon action by the wide range of statutory and voluntary agencies involved in dealing with the problem, it saw social services departments as the agency which should take the lead:

It will no doubt fall to social services authorities to draw together available information, initiate and co-ordinate action, and arrange for such guidance and preparation to be given to staff, volunteers and other helpers as may be necessary. The establishment of clear machinery at central and area level will facilitate the gathering and assessing of information about cases needing help and the co-ordination of the activities and resources of the statutory and voluntary agencies and workers involved. Where the circumstances of an elderly person are not already known to the social services authority, and visiting is therefore necessary, the authority will no doubt seek and receive the full co-operation of volunteer helpers through the voluntary bodies active in promoting the welfare of the elderly in their area. It may be found helpful to discuss with local officers of the Supplementary Benefits Commission, officers of housing, health and other local authority departments and representatives of local voluntary bodies, the strategy for tackling the problem and the role that each can best fulfil.[18]

A substantial section of the joint circular was concerned with improving the living conditions of the elderly: 'In many cases, comparatively minor work may effect considerable improvement − e.g. the installation of a new, alternative or additional heating appliance, draught exclusion or better insulation.' Appropriate action would depend on the tenure of the accommodation. Where the accommodation is owned by the local housing authority 'the social services authority will need to draw their attention to the situation so that they may take such action as they may consider appropriate.' In the case of private housing the approach of the circular was characterized by (an optimistic) reliance on voluntary effort and extreme caution about costs. 'In owner-occupied premises − subject always to the consent of the elderly person concerned − social services authorities may find it possible to enlist volunteers to undertake the necessary work provided the cost of materials can be met. Some owner-occupiers will be able to meet the cost themselves; in other cases local voluntary funds may be available; in others again the social services authority *may use its own powers* (our italics). In privately rented housing − where the consent of both the landlord and the elderly person would be necessary – volunteers might again undertake the work and either the landlord or tenant may be ready to meet the cost. Alternatively the other possibilities already mentioned would need to be investigated.'[19]

Whilst the circular did draw the attention of local authorities to the problems of the old and cold, and recognized the possibility that social services departments might use their own powers to alleviate them, it lacked any specific, detailed suggestions as to how departments might use these powers. With its concentration on voluntary help, and its references to the Supplementary Benefits Commission and housing departments, the circular shows the clear reluctance of the DHSS (and DOE) to encourage the widest possible use of social services departments' own powers and resources. However, the circular is important as a demonstration of concern about the 'old and cold' issue. This concern was underlined in September 1972 when the DHSS produced the explanatory leaflet 'Keeping Warm in Winter: simple guidance notes for those engaged in helping old people'. This leaflet, sent to all local authorities and widely circulated, was 'intended to suggest ways of making old people more comfortable during very cold weather by keeping them warm at the lowest possible fuel costs to themselves, and at the same time reducing personal danger from fire, explosion or asphyxiation.' It was primarily directed at 'volunteers with little or no knowledge of the subject', but 'it may also contain information of value to social workers.'

Social Services Departments: Policies and Practice

Our main concern in conducting this study was to discover what local authority social services departments were actually doing for the cold elderly. At the outset we visited a small number of local authority departments in order to discuss with practitioners the impressions we had gained from reading the available literature. We were also anxious to test the feasibility of collecting systematic information from a large number of authorities and consequently we took the opportunity of the visits to pilot a questionnaire. In the event, during the summer of 1974, we sent postal questionnaires to the 33 social services authorities in Greater London (32 boroughs plus the City). A more extensive survey of the authorities outside London was unfortunately not possible because of local government reorganization. A review of complementary health service provisions was also ruled out as our research period coincided with the immediate aftermath of the restructuring of the National Health Service.

Questionnaires were sent out in August 1974 and initially 30 of the 33 authorities completed them, 5 being accompanied by additional material.

This seemed a very high response rate given the recognized limitations of postal questionnaires and the general pressure under which social services departments were then operating. On the basis of these 30 replies we wrote a first draft report which was sent for comment to all the London boroughs. One further questionnaire was then received, together with a letter from another authority answering the main questions referred to in the circulated draft. The details outlined in the rest of this chapter relate, therefore, to the 32 of the 33 London authorities which eventually responded. A short article based on these findings,[20] together with a letter asking for comments, was subsequently sent to every social services department in the country outside London. A number of very useful and illuminating replies were received, and again, where appropriate, this information is referred to in the text.

A policy for the cold elderly?

One of our main concerns in undertaking the survey was to establish whether or not authorities had developed specific policies for dealing with the problem of the cold elderly. What kind of priority was generally afforded to this group? One possible indicator of the degree of importance attached to the issue by an authority was taken to be the degree of involvement of the social services committee in decisions about its prevention and treatment. Table 8.1 shows that the committees of 22 of the 32

Table 8.1

Social Services Committee Discussions

	Inner London	Outer London	All No.	%
Issue discussed by s.s. committee				
(April 1972 – October 1974)	7	15	22	69
Specific policies resulted	7	12	19	59
Total number of authorities in the study	13	19	32	100

respondents had discussed the problem between 1st April 1972 and 1st October 1974 and, in all but three of these, specific policies had resulted from the discussions.

Although two-thirds of London committees discussed the issue this may be more a reflection of the influence of central government prompting (the DHSS/DOE joint circular was issued in August 1972), than of local authorities' own priority commitments. Given that this lengthy circular with such wide implications was issued (and directed towards chief executives) it is perhaps more surprising that as many as one-third of London committees did not debate the cold elderly and their department's role in tackling the problem.

This is, of course, not to argue that an authority whose committee did not discuss hypothermia had no policy or provisions for the old and cold, or that those with active committees made adequate provisions. Indeed we discovered that, despite this fairly widespread formal recognition of the need to act, there was a considerable variation between authorities in the kinds of policies and practices they had developed. These can be seen by looking at local practices under four main headings: *administrative machinery; finance; information and advice;* and *services and facilities provided.*

Administrative machinery

What administrative arrangements had local authorities made, both internally and in the form of contact with other agencies? We asked departments whether they had established any special machinery to initiate or co-ordinate action in relation to the cold elderly, one of the recommendations of the joint circular. The results are presented in Table 8.2. Only 14 of the 32 respondents were found to have done so. Five departments had designated a responsible officer; 5 had established a working party of department officials and representatives of other agencies and

Table 8.2
Authorities Establishing Special Machinery

	Inner London	Outer London	All No.	All %
Type of machinery				
Designated SSD official	3	2	5	16
Joint committee	2	3	5	16
SSD Committee/Working party	—	2	2	6
Responsibility vested in existing section of SSD	—	1	1	3
No information	1	—	1	3
Special machinery established	6	8	14	44
Total number of authorities in the study	13	19	32	100

departments; 2 had set up a departmental working party or liaison committee; and one had specifically vested responsibility for the cold elderly
in an existing section of the department.

The picture was slightly more encouraging when we examined the
number of other agencies that each department had contacted in relation
to the cold elderly. The joint circular had specified the social services
departments' co-ordinating role, and Table 8.3 suggests that a number of
authorities had taken this very seriously and made contact with a wide
range of agencies.

Table 8.3
Departments or Agencies contacted about Hypothermia

	Inner London	Outer London	All No.	%
Local office of DHSS	11	16	27	87
One or more voluntary organizations	13	14	27	87
Borough housing department	11	10	21	68
Health department (Before 1st April 1974)	12	16	28	90
Area Health Authority	6	12	18	58
Executive Council (Before 1st April 1974)	1	6	7	23
Gas or Electricity Boards	2	3	5	16
GLC Housing department	1	1	2	—
Police	—	1	1	—
Total number of local authorities in the study	13	18	31*	

* One authority failed to answer this question.

The vast majority had been in contact with local DHSS offices, Health
Departments (prior to reorganization), and one or more voluntary organizations. Surprisingly perhaps, only just over half had so far contacted the
Area Health Authorities, whilst two-thirds had contacted the local housing department. Only 5 had entered into negotiations with the Gas or
Electricity Boards. Some authorities had contacted very few agencies or
other departments; some had obviously been involved in considerable
discussions across a wide field. Nine departments had contacted 3 or
fewer bodies; 8 had been in touch with 6 or more.

Finance

Specific expenditure is one very solid indication of the concern for, and
action on, the problem of the cold elderly. As can be seen from Table 8.4,

14 of the 32 departments earmarked a small proportion of their budget specifically for such expenditure, the amounts ranging from £800 to £4,300. In most cases, where we have the information, by far the largest amounts spent from this allocation were on heating appliances and adaptations.

Table 8.4

Authorities Earmarking Expenditure on the Cold Elderly

	Inner London	Outer London	All No.	All %
Part of budget earmarked	5	9	14	44
No special allocation	7	10	17	53
No information	1	—	1	3
All local authorities in the study	13	19	32	100

All the local authorities gave grants to local voluntary organizations concerned with the elderly, but only 14 were able to calculate exactly how much money this entailed. For these, the variation in the size of the grant was striking, ranging, for outer London boroughs, from £100 to £120,000 and for inner London from £250 to £150,000. Only one borough earmarked any part of this grant (£4,000 per annum) for expenditure on heating and insulation for the elderly, and (as reported above) part of this was specifically designated for payments to any elderly person in financial difficulty over heating costs.

Information and advice

Compared with, say, ten years ago the medical condition of hypothermia is now a widely recognized problem. Widespread, often greatly exaggerated publicity, has frequently thrust the issue before the public eye and made it an extremely emotive topic politically. However, awareness of the possibility of an acute medical condition and knowledge and information about how to prevent its occurrence, deal with it or even recognize it are rather different things. Social services department staff from field social workers to the far more numerous home helps and meals-on-wheel staff have frequent and continuous contacts with the elderly most at risk. Departments, therefore, have an important role to play by ensuring that their staff are adequately informed about the problems of the cold elderly and taught how to recognize signs of hardship and potential difficulty.

We asked departments to what extent the problem of hypothermia was being dealt with as part of its in-service training programmes for social workers and home helps, two of the groups most likely to be in contact with those at risk. The results are shown in Table 8.5.

Table 8.5

Hypothermia and In-service Training

	Home Helps	Social Workers
Referred to in passing	9	11
Specifically discussed	19	11
Not mentioned	2	7
No information	2	3
All local authorities in the study	32	32

As can be seen, home helps appear to receive rather more instruction on this problem than the social workers. In only 11 departments was hypothermia specifically discussed with social workers, in a further 11 it was referred to in passing and in 7 it was not discussed at all. However, in almost two-thirds of the authorities it was specifically discussed with home helps. In only one authority was there no specific mention of hypothermia in its training programmes for either social workers or home helps, but a further 8 included no more than a passing reference to it in the programmes for both groups. In only 8 was a specific discussion of hypothermia included in the training of both groups.

Authorities were asked if they had distributed any literature about hypothermia and/or the services available for tackling the problem (see Table 8.6).

Table 8.6

Hypothermia Information Distributed

	Inner London	Outer London	All No.	%
Information distributed to:				
The general public on request	9	8	17	53
The public by door-to-door distribution	1	4	5	16
Social work staff	9	14	23	72
Home helps	7	12	19	59
Other local authority staff	6	4	10	31
Number of departments distributing hypothermia literature to any group	10	16	26	81
Number of local authorities in the study	13	19	32	100

Six authorities had not distributed literature of any kind. Of the 26 who had, only 17 made literature available to the general public on request. Five departments had initiated a door-to-door distribution of information, 23 provided information for the social workers and 19 for home helps. It is perhaps interesting to note that as many as 15 authorities had given the problem sufficiently high priority to produce their own material explaining what the problem was and describing the services available for dealing with it. Some of them had developed their literature in conjunction with local voluntary organizations. Fourteen distributed DHSS material, including circulars and posters; 11 used literature produced by the local authority health departments; 4 used material produced by local voluntary organizations, and only 2 used material from the Health Education Council.

A number of social services departments from London and outside sent us copies of the literature prepared for distribution. These varied enormously in presentation and coverage. Some of them focused exclusively upon how to claim heating allowances or 'special help' from the Department of Health and Social Security, while others advised not only about financial help with heating costs, but how to keep warm, and deal with fuel emergencies. Several contained details of the address and telephone numbers of all the department's area offices, and one contained the plea: 'And *always* .... IF IN DOUBT.... ASK!' One non-London department, taking seriously its co-ordinating function, prepared and distributed 'packs' of available literature about hypothermia to 'identified leadership in the community', namely clergy, community groups, youth workers, neighbourhood and community workers, head teachers, social workers, health visitors and general practitioners(!). The pack contained a leaflet produced by the social services department itself, together with all the available DHSS literature, and material from Age Concern and other local authority departments. An even more ambitious experimental project was set up in Birmingham in the winter of 1975/6. For one month, Birmingham Social Services Department were to publicize a 'Daily Risk Warning' – 'an analysis of weather forecasts and environmental factors to predict the likely risks elderly people will face.'[21]

Departments were asked whether they had undertaken or sponsored any research relating to hypothermia and the cold elderly. The answers were somewhat disappointing in that only six authorities had established or supported any work of this kind. In three cases hypothermia was covered only incidentally as part of other research; three others focused specifically on the problem – one on the types of heating used by social services departments' clients, one on the heating needs of the elderly (conducted by school children) and one was a very competent review of research and a consideration of possible long-term policies for the authority.[22]

Services and facilities

What services and facilities were departments providing for the old and cold? All but one of the London authorities held stocks of heating appliances and aids, for distribution to the cold elderly at any time although three departments did not envisage drawing upon them except in fuel emergencies or exceptionally cold weather. Table 8.7 summarizes the main items stored.

Table 8.7
Types of Heating Appliances and Aids stocked by Departments

	Inner London	Outer London	All No.	%
Blankets	11	9	20	63
Electric blankets	8	10	18	56
Heating appliances	10	15	25	78
Hot water bottles	7	9	16	50
Thermos flasks	8	6	14	44
Nightwear	1	0	1	3
Clothes	3	1	4	13
Fuel	9	10	19	59
All local authorities in the study	13	19	32	100

There was great variation between authorities in their recorded stocks of appliances and aids. In outer London they ranged from one authority storing 6 bags of coal to another with 72 blankets, 12 electric blankets, 142 fires, 96 hot-water bottles and 36 thermos flasks. In inner London stocks were generally much larger, but even here the variation was considerable. One authority held 'several electric blankets', whilst another had 750 blankets, 86 electric blankets, 40 fires, 200 hot-water bottles, and 36 thermos flasks.

Table 8.8 provides an indication of the variety of heating appliances and aids held by the London authorities, but it should be treated with caution.

For example, one authority is credited with holding seven kinds of appliance or aid, a second only four. Examining the detailed holding of these authorities, however, one finds the first has 12 blankets, 6 electric blankets, 3 electric fires, 12 hot-water bottles, 12 flasks, 6 gas cylinder fires and 3 pairs of disposable gloves; the second has 1,035 blankets, 750 fires and provides clothing and fuel 'as necessary'.

Table 8.8

Variety of Stocks held*

	Inner London	Outer London	All	
			No.	%
None	0	1	1	2
One	1	3	4	13
Two/Three	3	9	12	38
Four/Five	3	4	7	22
Six/Seven	6	2	8	25
All local authorities in the study	13	19	32	100

* Figures refer to the following items: blankets, electric blankets, heating appliances, hot water bottles, thermos flasks, nightwear, clothes, fuel.

All of these figures on stocks of materials should be viewed with considerable caution, and some scepticism. As one London director was quick to point out, some authorities had obviously included in their returns the equipment held for the emergency services of fire, flood and disaster. In particular, large stocks are held for such emergencies by the 17 Thames-side authorities. Although these stocks would be available in a fuel emergency, the director argues, 'we certainly would not regard (them) as part of the cover for the elderly.' (For this reason, this department at least excluded from its returns the large emergency stocks held. Others may well have done the same.) This point was borne out by the amount of use made of stored equipment. Very few departments had made much use at all of their equipment during the previous admittedly 'mild' winter. Where any fires or blankets were issued they were in twos and threes rather than in any number. One authority was exceptional in that in the winter of 1973/4 it had used as many as 40 emergency fires and had 47 on long-term loan. Even this department had used only 15 blankets and one electric blanket.

A second point was raised by several directors who questioned the usefulness, when there are so many demands on a social services depart-ment's budget, of 'laying up stocks of equipment which could be bought at short notice anyway should the need arise'. Assuming that social services departments would indeed be able to acquire stocks at short notice at times of emergency or particular need, this point is valid if one assumes the role of the social services department is one of crisis intervention. If the adopted role were rather different — generally preventive, or concerned with relieving the discomfort due to the cold felt by so many elderly people

– presumably the approach to purchasing and using heating appliances and aids would also be rather different. At the very least it seems a useful question to ask why, when so many elderly people complain of feeling cold and of inadequate heating facilities, most London boroughs have large stocks of fires, blankets, electric blankets and so on which are rarely if ever put to use.

Concern about the elderly tends to be heightened during the coldest weather and during fuel crises of one kind or another. Our preliminary discussions with departments suggested that most authorities were likely to take special measures in these circumstances, and answers to our questions about stocks and use of heating appliances and aids confirmed our suspicion that response to major crises was for many the primary orientation. We asked authorities whether they had 'any specific plans for dealing with the cold elderly in the event of a fuel emergency or an exceptionally cold spell?' The answers are summarized in Table 8.9.

Table 8.9

Departmental Plans for Fuel Emergencies or Cold Spells

	Inner London	Outer London	All No.	%
Planned use of 'warmth centres' plus available blankets, heating appliances, etc.	3	3	6	19
Available blankets, heating appliances, etc.	6	10	16	50
Would make day care facilities available, but other supplies negligible	1	1	2	6
Few SSD supplies, but arrangements with local fuel merchants to ensure coal delivery to high priority cases	0	2	2	6
Departments with a contingency plan	10	16	26	81
Total number of LAs in the study	13	19	32	100

Twenty-six of the 32 authorities claimed to have developed specific plans for dealing with the cold elderly in the event of a fuel emergency. Six had no such plans. Provisions most commonly involved making available quantities of stored blankets and heating appliances, but a smaller number of departments had planned in addition to use 'warmth centres' to which the elderly could go during the day.

The cold elderly and the crisis approach

As we have seen there is evidence of considerable variation of attitudes and practice between departments. At one extreme there are those which take the problem extremely seriously in word and action and have made extensive contact with other agencies, have large numbers of aids and appliances and have done a great deal to spread awareness of the problem. A few have even organized research or mounted special action projects to deal with the problem of the cold elderly.

At the other extreme, there are a small number of apparently complacent authorities which seem to deny either that any such problem exists, or if it does that it is within the province of the social services department. These departments have few − if any − heating aids or appliances in stock, and in some cases have made no contingency plans for exceptionally cold spells or fuel emergencies. For these, hypothermia is seen as a medical condition and as such is the responsibility of the health authorities.

Across the centre of the spectrum are a very much larger group of authorities who adopt what might be termed a 'crisis approach' to the problem. They have taken to heart the existence of a severe medical condition known as hypothermia and have to a greater or lesser extent prepared plans for crises of different kinds when those 'at risk' may develop this condition.

It is of course true that during fuel or power crises, or in exceptionally cold weather, the problem will be that much worse and local authorities should gear themselves up to handle such emergencies − in fact most authorities did have contingency plans for this eventuality. The worry is that crisis thinking may prevent the adoption of strategies to deal with the more widespread problem − the day-to-day plight of the cold elderly: uncomfortable and unhappy, simply because they feel cold and live in cold surroundings.

Future policies

What policy implications emerge from this small inquiry? The very natural anxiety about the clinical condition of hypothermia and the attendant (exaggerated) publicity about the number of old people who die as a result has perhaps tended to draw attention away from what may now be considered to be a much greater problem, that of the miserably cold conditions in which millions of our elderly live. How can resources best be mobilized to produce warmer and more comfortable dwellings for Britain's old people? Clearly there is no single answer and any solution must involve several areas of social policy − many suggestions are made elsewhere in this book.

In the longer term we must hope − along with a number of directors of social services who wrote to us − that such miserable conditions can be prevented by better housing, with improved standards of insulation and central heating, and guaranteed rights to adequate pensions. In the shorter term, however, a number of services and agencies, both national and local, statutory and voluntary, will have to play a part in delivering a variety of services, aids, appliances and other forms of support.

Social services departments in particular, have a crucial role to play in protecting those at risk, preventing hardship, delivering services, educating staff and public about the problems, co-ordinating the agencies involved and, where necessary, referring critical cases to the medical authorities. Here, the Department of Health and Social Security could take a very much more positive line than in the past to assist local authorities to make an adequate response to the problem of the old and the cold. They should adopt a three-fold strategy.

First, the DHSS should encourage local authorities to redefine the narrowly conceived problem of hypothermia − a medical condition − as a more general problem of the cold elderly. In this way they could do a great deal to combat the crisis approach adopted by many local authorities.

Secondly, it should advise local authorities of the potential and the strengths of existing legislation. Much more extensive and imaginative use could be made of the powers which already exist. The Department should draw authorities' attention to the services, aids and appliances that can most effectively contribute to an attack on the problem. One director, for example, complained about the 'complete lack of technical advice from central government on appliances and appliance safety. An annual "Which?" type survey of equipment is badly needed.'

Finally, the Department should persuade, encourage or even cajole SSDs to adopt the recommendation of the 1972 Circular and establish machinery to initiate and co-ordinate action on the problem of the cold elderly. Someone, somewhere, has to take a lead. Once again the mantle of responsibility falls squarely across the already overburdened shoulders of the local authorities' social services departments.

Policy

Chapter 9
Housing and Heating

In simple terms an end to the problem of the old and cold – or certainly a large part of that problem – depends on there being adequately heated housing available for all old people. A straightforward objective, but one that begs many questions: what standards of heating are necessary to achieve warm conditions?; are such standards being achieved for new housing construction?; and, for older accommodation, i.e. most housing, how can standards be increased? (how is improvement policy contributing to this?); what role can be played by home insulation?; are the elderly benefiting as much as others from the growing public and official interest in insulation?; how can housing authorities improve thermal conditions in publicly owned accommodation?; can elderly tenants be enabled to afford to use the heating equipment that is provided?; how should heating be paid for in council housing?; should district heating be developed in the future?; can housing management practices and policies (particularly those concerned with allocation) be made more sensitive to the 'old and cold' question? These are the main questions that will be discussed in this chapter, some of which concern the possibility of improving the situation of the elderly in the short-to-medium term, while others have long-term implications.

Heating Standards

In the longer term one of the major attacks on the problem of cold conditions must be through steadily improving standards of heating and insulation. Such improvements are, of course, useless unless better heating can be paid for. Questions of cost are discussed later in this chapter, while the implications for our social security policies are discussed in Chapter 7. But what do we mean by improved heating? And what insulation standards are necessary today and for the future?

There is a great deal of room for improvement as our own survey results show (see Chapter 4). Most of Britain's old people have room temperatures below recommended levels and substantial numbers have extremely cold homes. Only 24% of our sample had central heating. The heating standards of the old are worse than those of the population generally, but even so the main problem is likely to be one of outdated heating methods that, while changing, are often ill-suited to modern needs in general and inefficient for providing for adequate warmth in particular.

It is regrettable, but not surprising, that concern about heating in Britain has been most evident at times of energy crises, rather than as a result of positive planning or anxiety about cold conditions. In recent years, for example, promotion of heating and energy into an important policy issue results from the action of oil sheikhs and not from mounting evidence about the plight of the 'old and cold'.

Similar concerns were evident during and after the Second World War. One of the most important documents on heating standards was published in 1945.[1] The Egerton Report discussed heating questions in a way which has probably not been matched for thoroughness since. The report commented that, partly due to a supply of 'cheap and abundant coal', the ordinary person has seldom adopted a critical attitude towards the appliances he uses and the building he lives in.' However, the situation had changed and prices were rising and so 'there is ample incentive to the adoption of more efficient and economical methods of heating.'[2]

The report made suggestions about desirable temperature levels, but not before noting that:—

> It is notoriously difficult to define the basic human needs for warmth, and every pronouncement made, by however eminent an authority, is liable to arouse controversy.[3]

For living-rooms it was noted that 'an equivalent air temperature of about 65°F has generally been considered a suitable standard for this country for warmth when sitting for lengthy periods.' It noted that most people feel comfortably warm within the range 62–66°F equivalent temperature and that the variation should not generally exceed the range 60–68°F 'for the upper and lower limits will present rather extreme conditions.'[4]

The report of 1945 also discussed the heating of bedrooms and noted that there was 'some conflict of opinion as to whether in the ordinary way bedrooms should be heated, provided sufficient bed clothes are available.' However, the committee concluded that:—

'The disadvantages of the completely unheated room, however, are so considerable that there can be little real doubt on the matter'.[5]

The report felt that facilities should be provided for obtaining an equivalent temperature of 50°–55°F during dressing and undressing when the room is occupied during the day and for preventing the temperature from falling below 45°–50°F during the night. Also, in case of illness, at least one bedroom should be capable of being warmed up to 65°F.

The report of the Egerton Committee is interesting and of significance for several reasons. Set up in 1942, and reporting in 1945, it represents a bold and imaginative attempt at war-time social planning. No equivalent appraisal of this subject has been attempted in more than 30 years since it was produced. Its concern to foster a 'critical attitude' towards heating and its anxiety about rising costs serves to remind us that the Western world's concern about energy in the mid-70s is not totally without precedent. It can also be noted that the temperature levels recommended by the committee over three decades ago are still not being experienced by large numbers of today's elderly.

It is also of interest to look at some evidence about heating habits during the war and in the early post-war period. This is possible because of a series of surveys conducted by the Wartime Social Survey and its successor. Not merely of historic interest, a brief description of some main findings helps us to appraise contemporary standards and, perhaps, to appreciate the attitudes of today's elderly towards heating (their current heating habits being, in part, determined by earlier experience).

In February and March of 1942 the Wartime Social Survey interviewed over 5,000 households in the 'lower paid section of the working class'.[6] The major findings of this inquiry related to the restrictive use of heating. One room only was heated in about 74% of all households and 'bedrooms were not heated in nearly 87% of all households on both week-days and Sundays.'[7] A Social Survey carried out in 1948/49 interviewed 2,600 households using a general population sample.[8] This is principally interesting for the snapshot picture it produces of the heating appliances in use at this time. It showed that 96% had open coal fires in the main living-room; 2%, 'other' coal fires; 5%, electric fires; 2%, gas fires; and only 1%, central or district heating.[9] The report noted, however, that 'it is quite likely that changes are taking place rapidly in the heating habits of the people of this country.'[10]

Another Social Survey inquiry was carried out in 1952.[11] This provides more evidence about the use of heating. It found that 68% of the 'general sample' had no bedrooms heated 'at least once a week in winter' and the proportion among those in post-war local authority housing was 40%.[12] Thus, while more people were heating their bedrooms in the early 50s than was the case in the middle of the war, the proportions were still generally low. These results provide an interesting background against which to consider the results to similar questions asked in our own survey (see Chapter 6).

How warm do houses need to be? As the Egerton Committe noted there will be no one, authoritative answer to this question. For while there will be temperature levels that are so low that life is endangered, it is more difficult to pronounce on the temperature that is required to maintain comfortable conditions. In practice, ideas about what such conditions are will change with time, will vary from country to country (expectations are very high in North America for example) and will reflect economic conditions and increasing aspirations. But what is the current position?

In 1961 the Parker Morris Report was published.[13] This report argued that: 'better heating is the key to the design of homes at the present time' and that there was 'an increasing demand for higher comfort levels'. It noted that 'The person moving into a new home increasingly expects to be *warm*. In factory and office such a standard is usually taken for granted, and the expectation is spreading to the home.'[14] Regarding standards, the report recommended that the minimum should be an installation capable of heating the kitchen and the areas used for circulation to 55°F and the living areas to 65°F (when the outside temperature is 30°F). It also recommended that where families require the use of bedrooms (as studies or bed-sitting rooms) a more expensive installation capable of heating the bedrooms to 65°F would represent the greater value for money.[15]

In 1969 the then Ministry of Housing and Local Government issued a circular on housing 'specially designed for, and intended for occupation by, old people'.[16] This laid down a mandatory, minimum standard of an installation capable of maintaining a temperature of 21°C (70°F) in the living area, bathroom, hall or lobby, bedroom and kitchen.

This official recognition of the elderly's need for adequate heating standards also came from the Department of the Environment's Housing Directorate which noted in 1973 that: 'older persons need higher temperatures for comfortable living conditions.'[17]

The Department of Health and Social Security also supported this call for higher temperatures. In 'Keeping Warm In Winter' the Department advised:—

> To keep old people warm in winter the living room temperature should be about 70°F when the temperature outside is 30°F. Bathrooms and bedrooms should be kept at the same temperature if possible, but in any event should be kept warm.[18]

It is unfortunate that this leaflet has now been withdrawn and '. . . the DHSS no longer recommends 70°F nor any other temperature'.[19]

One reason for the DHSS's change of mind appears to be because 'there is no medical evidence to show that elderly people need higher temperatures than anyone else.'[20]

This is an extraordinary argument. While it may be right, as the DHSS also argued, that no evidence points to a precise temperature that old people require to maintain health (nor could it, as needs vary), there is massive evidence about the risks faced by the elderly. The suspicion must exist that the DHSS is using a narrow technical argument to withdraw a recommended temperature level which our own survey results and other evidence shows is not being achieved by the vast majority of old people in Britain.

What kind of heating is being provided for new housing? A comprehensive picture is not available, but we do have data for new local authority and new town accommodation. For several years now more than 90% of new local authority accommodation in England and Wales has been provided with central heating.[21]

The trend towards central heating is to be generally welcomed. Our own evidence supports its value. Central heating results in higher room temperatures than those produced by other forms of heating. Thus it is one of the most obvious preventive measures that can and should be taken. However, there is an important caution. Central heating is an expensive piece of technology that cannot be lightly exchanged for other forms of heating and it is not always easily converted for use by alternative fuels. Indeed, many households – including many council tenants – have no choice over their heating methods and have to rely on a certain form of central heating. This may produce particular problems. For example, following the Ronan Point disaster many tall blocks of flats have only electrical central heating installed in them for reasons of safety. This form of heating is now very expensive. Should the costs of this policy decision lie where they fall[22] – with the tenant; or should the public (whose representatives made the decision about the type of heating and the type of housing) pay some of the cost – for all or some of the tenants? Questions concerning payment are discussed later.

Having discussed new building, we now need to consider the existing housing stock. What are the problems here? There can be little doubt that many old people have inadequate heating appliances. Our survey results demonstrate the importance of central heating and yet only 24% of the sample had central heating.[23] At present there is no obvious way of ensuring that an old person in need of adequate heating equipment can receive it. As is noted in Chapter 7, supplementary benefits officers can award an exceptional needs payment for the repair or replacement of an ineffective appliance, but this power is not used a great deal and is, in any case, not likely to be the most effective way of tackling the issue. As we noted in Chapter 8, local authority social services departments can supply heating appliances and, while most of the London social services departments stock them, little use seems to be made of this equipment. It would seem sensible to regard the power of both the Supplementary Benefits Commission and local social services departments as essentially emergency or back-up provisions. But they will need to be more extensively used unless 'mainstream' provision comes from somewhere.

In the longer term, one must look towards housing improvement policy as the means by which existing housing should be adequately heated. Under the 1974 Housing Act a 'grant towards the cost of space heating up to Parker Morris standards may reasonably be given when this forms part of the cost of a scheme for converting a property into flats or for the comprehensive improvement of a dwelling.' However, the Department of the Environment guidance is that 'grant should not be given for the installation of central heating, either on its own or linked with other inessential improvements.'[24]

Insulation

In the early 1970s the importance of insulation became more and more recognized. The government's 'Save It' campaign recommended insulation. Do-it-yourself and Sunday colour magazines wrote about it, standards were raised and thousands of owner-occupiers up and down the country eagerly, if uncomfortably, unrolled or scattered appropriate insulating material in their lofts. Though the recognition of the importance of insulation has been rapid, even now it is far from complete and in any case is unlikely to help those most in need.

As A. W. Pratt has said, insulation is an important way of achieving recommended temperature levels. The alternative is to rely on the householder to burn a greater amount of fuel.

> In this country the latter approach is preferred and has yielded an almost bewildering assortment of appliances and systems of space heating encouraged by the major fuel industries and with seemingly little consideration for economy in the use of fuel.[25]

The case for insulation can be summed up by quoting the words of one authority, written 30 years ago:—

> It is not enough only to provide domestic appliances which use the fuel efficiently in the production of heat. It is important also to ensure that the heat so obtained is not unnecessarily dissipated and wasted. In the past, insufficient attention has been given in Great Britain to the improvements that can be effected by the judicious use of insulating material and to the design and construction of houses, taking overall costs into account, to prevent unnecessary loss of heat to the atmosphere.[26]

This quotation also shows that concern about insulation is no new phenomenon. Indeed the Egerton Report of 1945 noted that 'in most European countries great importance is attached to the proper insulation of houses'[27] and called for more attention to be given to the conservation of heat in the building of houses. However it was not really until another 30 years later that government began to take the need for adequate standards of insulation seriously.

Costs and savings

There is no doubt that a great deal of warmth is lost from British homes. The National Consumer Council notes that 'as a rough generalisation three-quarters of the heat produced in a semi-detached house is wasted. Of this, about 35 per cent is lost through the cavity walls, 25 per cent through the roof, 15 per cent through the floor, 15 per cent by draughts and 10 per cent through the windows. A well-insulated house would lose only a quarter of heat produced.'[28]

The Building Research Establishment (BRE) has produced a thorough review and analysis of the whole field of energy saving in housing. The report showed that space heating in the approximately 19 million dwellings in the United Kingdom represented about 16 per cent of the 'national primary energy consumption' – 'or as much as the whole transport sector'.[29]

The BRE report demonstrates that calculating savings from thermal insulation or other energy conservation measures is no easy matter. One problem, for example, is the fact that many people in poorly heated dwellings prefer increased warmth to the savings on fuel that could be achieved (and hence one needs to distinguish between theoretical and actual savings). Nevertheless the report is in no doubt on the basic issue that a great deal of energy can be saved by insulating houses:—

> Thermal insulation saves energy irrespective of how the space heating is supplied and is also important to thermal comfort. If the existing housing stock had been cavity-filled where possible, if the loft insulation had been improved, and windows double-glazed, the UK energy consumption would have been 3 to 4 per cent less taking account of the past evidence that some of the potential fuel saving in older properties with only partial heating would have been taken up in increased comfort. If the full potential had been realised the energy savings would have been about 5 per cent'.[30]

Establishing that energy savings can be made, however, is only a first step. Cost-effectiveness is a crucial issue. Is it actually worth spending

scarce resources on thermal insulation? An answer to this question
depends, in part, on future real increases in the cost of energy. Accordingly the BRE analysis is based on three alternative hypotheses. The
current cost hypothesis assumes that in the long run there would be no
further increase in real terms in the cost of energy after January 1975. The
second hypothesis assumes an annual real increase of 4 per cent per
annum and the third an annual rise of 7 per cent (i.e. doubling every 10
years). Bearing this factor in mind the BRE study's conclusions included
the following:—

> . . . cavity fill and loft insulation are cost-effective at current cost for a dwelling
> heated to a good standard of comfort with good controls. For new constructions
> the measure is likely to be cost-effective at current costs even if some of the
> savings are likely to be taken up in improved thermal comfort. For other
> dwellings with cavity walling the measure is cost-effective at about the 4 per cent
> fuel cost profile. Loft insulation of the remainder of the dwellings by contractors
> is marginally cost-effective at current costs though certainly cost-effective at
> current costs if the householder undertakes the installation himself. Double
> glazing is not cost-effective at any of the fuel cost profiles except in the case of a
> well heated, well controlled dwelling where it is just about cost-effective at the
> severest fuel cost profiles.[31]

Standards

The development of insulation standards can be briefly noted. The trans-
mittance or 'U' value of a construction is defined as the amount of heat
energy conducted through unit area of the construction in unit time with
unit air temperature difference between the two sides. The lower the 'U'
value, the lower is the heat loss through the building surface.* In this
section values for roof or loft insulation will be given by way of illustration.

It is only comparatively recently that government has laid down
minimum standards for thermal insulation. Before 1965 local authorities
made their own regulations, guided by the 1953 Model Byelaws on Building issued by the Ministry of Housing. These recommended a 'U' value of
(not more than) 2.38. This was amended in 1959 to not more than 1.42, the
equivalent to 1 inch of lagging.

In 1965 minimum requirements for England and Wales were set out in
the Building Regulations. These confirmed a 'U' value of 1.42 (1.13 for
Greater London). Under the 1963 Building Standards (Scotland) Regulations the 'U' value was 1.13.

---

*'U' values were formerly measured by the imperial unit, i.e. Btu/ft²h deg. F. The SI unit is
now used, i.e. W/m^2 deg. C., and is the one referred to in the text.

These recommended minima were low by any standard. The Egerton Report of 1945 had recommended a 'U' value of 1.13 and had noted that 'still lower values are to be preferred when they can be obtained economically'.[32] It is certainly the case that most of the rest of Europe has taken the need for insulation far more seriously than Britain. During most of the post-war period, this country has been near to the bottom of the European ladder as far as insulation is concerned.

The dramatic rise in energy costs has brought about a change in official attitudes. Since January 1975, Building Regulations have required a 'U' value of 0.6, the equivalent of two inches of insulating material. This is the standard for both new construction and improvements.[33] The 'Save It' campaign went further, however, and recommended a three- or four-inch layer of loft insulation.[34]

Insulating older dwellings

Concern about insulation standards is usually focused on new dwellings, but progress in this direction is only one way of improving the thermal insulation of Britain's housing, and it is very slow. In the period 1970–76 an average of approximately 316,000 new dwellings have been built in Great Britain each year[35] (and this annual total represents less than 2% of the housing stock). Even more important therefore than the right standards for new housing is the improvement of the existing stock. The scope and potential here is tremendous. It is estimated that some 6–8 million dwellings have cavity walls that could be filled.[36] Eight million dwellings, with suitable access, have no loft insulation and two-thirds of those with loft insulation have less than the recommended minimum of 3 inches. 3½ million homes with tanks suitable for lagging have none and three-quarters of existing lagging is less than the recommended minimum of 3 inches.[37] How can the desired improvement be carried out?

The provision of adequate insulation in existing homes poses different problems both within and between tenure groups. At one extreme the problem may be fairly easy to solve. Many younger owner-occupiers have already insulated the lofts of their houses and many more can be encouraged to do so in the future, spurred on by the right sort of government-sponsored publicity and features in newspapers and magazines. Such owner-occupiers can be persuaded of the economic advantages of roof insulation, many can find the necessary cash to purchase the materials and most will be fit and agile enough to carry out the job for themselves. At the other extreme, however, is the aged widow living on her own in physically inadequate privately rented accommodation. Her landlord may not be easily persuaded to insulate, especially as he will probably not be paying for the heat lost through the roof. The tenant herself may not be able to afford it and will certainly not be able to lay the material down. In any case she will be less likely to find out about the advantages of insulation.

In between these two extremes there will be a variety of circumstances and, in many, it will not be easy to ensure adequate insulation. For example many owner-occupiers are elderly and may well not be able to insulate their homes for themselves. Many such owners will be poor – approximately one in six supplementary pensioners are owner-occupiers[38] – and unable to afford insulating materials. The position of local authority tenants may not be much brighter, for local councils may not consider insulation a priority.

The need for insulation now features as an aspect of government improvement policy. Since 1975 the equivalent of a two-inch layer of insulating material has been a requirement for obtaining the full standard for an intermediate grant. This will not generally qualify for exchequer grant aid, however, except where the authority considers it to be in the interest of an elderly or disabled tenant.[39] The aid would normally be at the rate of 50% but could be as high as 90% in general improvement or housing action areas. Unfortunately the implementation of this provision has been a disappointment and few elderly people have benefited under it so far.[40]

What can be done to ensure that the elderly and other groups in need are able to have their homes adequately insulated? There is a unique opportunity here, for while the successful attack on the twin problems of hypothermia and cold conditions depends mainly on the development of mainstream housing, social security and other programmes, an insulation campaign presents a direct way of helping the old and cold. Furthermore the right sort of policy would meet both social and economic needs. What is required is a campaign and programme that would identify those most in need of insulation and then provide appropriate help (ranging from straightforward draught-proofing to more sophisticated work) using as manpower unemployed construction workers and unemployed youth. Such a programme would, of course, be expensive but, by utilizing the labour of the unemployed, savings would be made on unemployment and supplementary benefit. Also, over time, the programme would make a good deal of economic sense through reductions in fuel costs.

Such a programme would need to be carefully planned centrally (involving the collaboration of the Department of Employment, Department of Energy and the Department of Environment and other agencies); it would involve the full participation of the local authorities, and the active co-operation of voluntary bodies (to help identify those in need) and the trade unions.

In fact some work along these lines has already been carried out under the Job Creation Programme. By the end of June 1977 86 local authorities were involved in schemes in which over 80,000 houses had been insulated at a total cost approaching £1 million.[41]

Prompted by a report of the Child Poverty Action Group and the Research Institute for Consumer Affairs,[42] the Department of the Environment mounted an experimental heating project for the elderly.[43] The aim of the project was to carry out low-cost improvement to the homes of old people with the help of three local authorities. Typical improvements carried out included draught-proofing of doors and windows, and replacement of inefficient heaters.

The project can be regarded as a success in that most of the old people reported feeling warmer after the improvements had been carried out, although some temperatures were still below current standards. The insulation work in this project was relatively inexpensive – about £40 per dwelling for draught-proofing and roof insulation at about £30.

A national programme of this kind, providing that it is carried out with flexibility and imagination, could make a major impact on aspects of the problem of the old and cold. But one should not pretend that this provides the whole solution. It is likely, for example, that improvements will often be hard to achieve in the privately rented housing sector, and ultimately warm and comfortable housing will require general housing improvements and not just minor work designed to improve thermal insulation.[44]

District Heating[45]

District heating is 'the piped distribution of heat, using the medium of hot water, to all categories of buildings in towns for space and water heating.'[46] Such a scheme replaces the need for a proliferation of individual boilers, tanks, chimneys and other equipment for space and water heating purposes. District heating schemes vary a great deal. In the UK most of the schemes are group heating schemes of typically 100–200 houses, but some quite large networks exist, for example in Nottingham (City centre and 7,000 houses) and Peterborough (3,500).

District heating is in much greater evidence in some other countries. In Denmark there are some 460 different schemes and 30% of domestic heat is supplied by 'district heating – large schemes including combined heat and power CHP' (and a further 23% by 'group heating schemes'). In Sweden some 20% of space and water heating is supplied through district heating schemes and in Germany the proportion is expected to reach 12% by 1980.[47]

The advantages of district heating have been noted by many.[48] Ernest Haseler has argued that the system is 'the logical development of the idea behind central heating'.[49] Haseler, a leading authority on the subject, has advocated district heating on grounds of economy, efficiency and comfort and argues that:—

> District heating fits the bill perfectly whether supplying warm air heaters, radiators or embedded panels, and heating of bedrooms is at very little extra cost. There is no smell, noise, fire, shock, explosion or asphyxiation hazard or the possibility of condensation in the home.[50]

District heating has received some encouragement from government. In a 1971 circular the Department of the Environment noted that:—

> Many local authorities have already installed district heating in their new housing schemes. Some of the very successful ones have been for comparatively small numbers of dwellings, such as accommodation specially designed for old people, but district heating seems particularly suitable for large developments and the Secretaries of State encourage local authorities to consider the applicability of district heating at an early stage of their thinking.[51]

Despite these arguments, however, district heating has not yet made a substantial impact on Britain. It is estimated that, in the UK, less than 1% of the space heating load is supplied by district heating schemes,[52] and provisional figures for 1975 show that only 4.5% of new local authority housing include district heating, the figures for 1972, 1973 and 1974 being 10.9%, 9.6% and 8.1% respectively.[53]

The debate

A thorough analysis of the arguments for and against district heating supplied from combined heat and power (CHP) stations was presented by a group of experts in a 1977 Department of Energy report. The general principle in favour of district heating was accepted:—

> It is inherent in the method of producing electricity from a normal power station that only about one-third of the energy content of the input fuel is converted to electricity. The remaining two-thirds is discharged mainly in lukewarm water to cooling towers, rivers or the sea. By changing the operation of the station to combined heat and power (CHP) production, hot rather than lukewarm water can be produced. This may reduce the electricity production somewhat but, because the heated water is now available at a useful temperature, the overall efficiency with which the input fuel is used can be greatly increased, provided, of course, that uses are found for the very large quantities of hot water.[54]

There is therefore no doubt about the basic advantage of CHP district heating, that is its conservation of energy. However 'the real question is whether it can do so economically'[55], and this proves to be a very difficult question to answer. The Department of Energy working party's economic analysis depends on judgments about a number of complex questions concerning the future. These are (1) the availability and price of different fuels in the future compared with other goods; (2) standards of heating and thermal insulation; (3) sighting policy on nuclear and conventional power stations; (4) future living patterns and housing densities; (5) views about the foregoing of present benefits for 'less certain, but perhaps more substantial benefits in the long term'.[56]

The report's main conclusion presents a less enthusiastic picture of district heating than emerges from some earlier writing:—

With present fuel prices and fuel availability, and with a test discount of 10% there is no economic incentive to introduce CHP and district heating except in particular circumstances. It would be definitely uneconomic in most cases for the conversion of existing cities, though it may be economic in limited high density areas within those cities.[57]

The report also discusses a longer-term view. At the turn of the century natural gas and oil will be becoming scarce and expensive and in these circumstances CHP/district heating would be economically attractive compared to either direct electric heating or gas produced from coal. Other possibilities for heating exist but there are many uncertainties about these. The report argues that:—

... around the turn of the century, there is likely to be a good economic case for the large scale exploitation of CHP/district heating in large cities.[58]

Timing is crucial, the report argues, and 'if we wait we may well close the CHP option to our regret.' It therefore advocates the selection of a pilot city for the planning and implementation of CHP and warns that: 'Without strong government initiatives CHP will not develop to any significant extent in the UK.'[59]

District heating is a complex subject. Much depends on the economics of such schemes. If, for example, a lower test discount rate had been adopted by the Department of Energy working party, district heating would appear as a more attractive prospect. Looking into the future – into the post North Sea oil period – it is likely that district heating will become more popular and necessary. The need to start now on one or more pilot projects is therefore essential.

Heating Costs

It was argued in Chapter 6 that the cost of heating is a major problem for many of the elderly and, in many cases, is likely to be a direct cause of cold housing. Family Expenditure Survey data support this contention (see Chapter 2) as does our own survey evidence. Two-thirds of our respondents found heating 'rather expensive' (Table 6.8) and, of those who wanted more heat in the house (Table 6.9) the vast majority (88%) gave expense as the reason why they did not have more.

Since our national survey was conducted (1972) there have been major increases in the cost of heating. If the old were worried about heating costs then, and were cold as a result, the position today must be substantially worse. Heating costs (and the issues related to them) are a large and complex subject. It is worthy of a major study in its own right and, indeed, there have been several reports dealing with aspects of this question in recent years.[60] But here it is only possible to consider briefly increases in costs to consumers and to review the important related issues of pricing policies, subsidies and disconnection.

Costs and prices

Heating costs have increased a great deal in recent years. The National Consumer Council has summarized the position as follows:—

> Although price rises had in general been accelerating in the seven years up to 1973, the beginning of 1974 marked a sharp change in the trend for fuel prices, with an increase of 25% in 1974 compared with only 6% the year before. In 1975 prices rose 7 times as steeply as they did in 1966 – by 35% for fuel and 23¹/₂% for all items. Before 1974, fuel prices on the whole rose less than prices in general; in 1974 and 1975 fuel prices rose considerably more.[61]

The impact on the consumer of these percentage increases was obviously considerable. Thus, the old lady who paid 21p for a gallon of paraffin in January 1974, paid 37p in January 1976 and 46¹/₂p in June 1977. To take another example, standard rate electricity (p/KWh) averaged 0.95p in January 1974, 1.95p in January 1976 and 2.36p in June 1977.

There are two main causes for these huge price increases. The first is the general increase in energy costs that have occurred in the mid-1970s. The second is the ending of price restraint and, consequently, the removal of government subsidies for gas and electricity.

Social costs

The rapid increase in heating costs has a number of implications for social policy in the broadest sense. One of these is conservation. Energy is not only becoming more expensive, it is also getting scarce. And while Britain's position is relatively better than that of many other countries, the conservation of energy is as important here as elsewhere. Adequate domestic insulation is one aspect and its implications for the elderly were discussed earlier. Another implication of increased heating costs concerns their impact on different groups of consumers. How does pricing policy affect the poor?

Pricing policy

The relationship between energy costs and pricing policy of the gas and electricity industries is crucial to the heating needs of the elderly. The issue has been treated at some length in several recent reports and it is useful here to pinpoint the basic issue by noting the findings of the National Consumer Council. Having reviewed the two types of domestic electricity tariff and the three domestic gas tariffs, their report notes that 'smaller consumers pay a higher average price per unit for fuel than larger ones.' The Council explored the implications of this for the poor and concluded that:—

> ... the great majority of low income households were small consumers and would benefit from a flat rate tariff with no standing charge, under which small and large consumers would pay the same average price per unit. Though a minority of poorer households who are relatively large consumers would be harmed by the change, there are a number of ways in which the harm could be offset.[62]

A related issue of great importance concerns the method of payment – e.g. pre-payment meters, easy payment schemes, collection with rent – for inadequate and insensitive practice here can greatly exacerbate the hardship problem caused by increasing costs.[63] The Supplementary Benefits Commission has commented that:—

> It is an unfortunate piece of timing that the rise in fuel prices has been accompanied by the decline of the coin-in-the-slot 'pre-payment' meter and its replacement by the 'credit meter' which advertises its existence only once a quarter or so. It is in many ways remarkable that a country which largely still pays its benefits and its wages weekly should have debated so little a process which meant that people were going to have to budget for a significant part of their expenditure over 13 weeks.[64]

In principle, for local authority and housing association tenants, the ideal arrangement is probably the payment of a fixed sum for heating with the rent. In practice there are different sorts of schemes, but the most ambitious was probably the one operated in Birmingham. Under this scheme elderly council tenants spread their fuel costs over a year by paying a fixed, regular amount with the rent. The Corporation then paid for heating, even if consumption had been more than had been allowed for. The advantages of the scheme were: that it allowed the tenant to pay for heating at frequent intervals; adequate heating without the fear of huge bills; and the SBC's recognition of this scheme which pays exceptional circumstances additions for costs over and above the notional amount in the scale rates (see Chapter 7). However, the scheme did have certain disadvantages. Individual elderly tenants might have felt, for example, that they could spend less on heating than specified by the Corporation under the scheme and yet not have the opportunity to do so. But it was the sheer cost of the scheme for the Corporation that eventually brought about a drastic revision. The first year of the scheme cost Birmingham £750,000 and forced the Corporation to increase the charges drastically, and consequently participating tenants have declined from 21,000 to just over 12,000. And in 1977 the SBC decided to withdraw support from the scheme.[65]

Meeting Social Need

Government has not devised an appropriate strategy for tackling the hardships caused to those most in need by the increase in heating costs. Instead it has reacted in a number of piecemeal ways. One such way, the expansion of supplementary benefit heating additions, was discussed in Chapter 7. Others concern the problem of disconnections and the rapid increase in electricity costs.

Disconnections

A great deal of attention has been focused in recent years on the problem of fuel disconnections for non-payment. The number of disconnections has certainly increased in the wake of price increases. Gas disconnections totalled 32,934 in 1972/3 and 39,842 in 1975/6 (for Great Britain). Electricity disconnections totalled 117,369 in 1972/3 and an estimated 138,399 in 1975/6 (for England and Wales).

While these numbers are small in proportion to total consumers (representing 0.37% of gas consumers in 1975/6 and 0.8% of electricity consumers)[66], for those affected, disconnections represent major social problems and the NCC has estimated that 'perhaps 25,000 households are without electricity or gas at any one time.'[67] Apart from the NCC Report the issue has been extensively discussed in the Oakes Report[68]; the report of the Select Committee on Nationalised Industries[69]; and by organizations such as CPAG[70] and the British Association of Settlements.[71]

In December 1976 the Gas and Electricity Industries published a code of practice 'designed to protect genuine hardship cases from disconnection'.[72] One of the main purposes of the code is to give certain protection to four categories of possible hardship, viz. recipients of supplementary benefits; recipients of family incomes supplement; the unemployed; and families with children under the age of 5 years. In these cases it is hoped that the local social security office or social services department will become involved.

Direct payment

As noted in Chapter 7 exceptional needs payments (ENPs) can be paid to supplementary benefit recipients to meet fuel debts. Since February 1976 the Supplementary Benefits Commission has introduced a new procedure for cases of fuel debts. This applies when it is felt that an ENP is not justified, but where hardship would be caused by disconnection (generally, in households with young children, the old or the sick). If the debt cannot be paid from savings or by help from earning non-dependants, the social security office can pay part of the weekly benefit direct to the gas or electricity board. The aim of this procedure is 'to ensure that the claimant pays for his current consumption, to reduce the debt over a period, and to avert disconnection'.

A not dissimilar 'savings deduction' scheme is also in operation. Designed to help claimants with budgeting, it involves keeping back some of each week's benefit and returning it to the supplementary benefit recipient when the fuel bill has to be paid. Both the above schemes affect only a small number of supplementary pensioners, but are used much more for non-pensioner claimants. In December 1976 a total of 48,000 supplementary benefit claimants were participating in the two schemes for electricity bills (of whom 6,000 were pensioners). The respective figures for gas were 21,000 and 3,000.

The £25 million scheme

Another piecemeal policy was the decision in 1976 to allocate £25 million to help those 'likely to have the greatest difficulty with fuel bills' in the winter of 1976/77. The aim of the scheme was to reduce the electricity bills of recipients of supplementary benefits and family income supplement by 25% for a period of one quarter.[73] Quite apart from its inevitable stop-gap nature, one inevitable drawback to the scheme was the difficulty of publicizing it to all potential recipients and there has been a low take-up rate.

Housing Needs and Policy

So far in this chapter, we have discussed various issues that relate directly to heating, but the successful attack on cold conditions does not just depend (indeed, does not primarily depend) on specific policies to tackle this problem, but rather on mainstream policies and services. What does this mean in the field of housing? We can only briefly explore this question here.

In Chapter 2 the housing circumstances of Britain's Elderly were reviewed. It was shown that the old generally live in poorer accommodation than the rest of the population. A change in this position is likely to have a powerful impact on cold conditions. However, when discussing the housing needs of the elderly, one major pitfall should be avoided. This is to consider the aged as a homogenous group. For as the Cullingworth report observed:— 'the elderly differ as much as the non-elderly in their housing conditions, needs and aspirations.'[74]

To ignore this can easily lead the policy-maker into proposing uniform and inappropriate measures. This outlook, allied to that which considers old age itself a problem, can in particular lead to an emphasis on specialized accommodation for the elderly which is likely in practice to be appropriate for only a minority.

Indeed, it is something of a paradox that, while most interest has been focused on special housing for the elderly – sheltered housing for example – it is manifestly apparent that most old people will never inhabit such accommodation and indeed most would prefer not to. Although the statistics need to be interpreted carefully, it is noteworthy that 70% of our national sample said that they were 'completely satisfied' with their accommodation. And it is officially recognized that:—

> old people prefer to live, and benefit from living, as independently as possible, and therefore, in particular, in housing in the community rather than in hospitals or residential homes.[75]

What are the implications of this? One of the most important concerns the conditions of housing.

Housing conditions

In 1976 an estimated 794,000 dwellings in England were still 'unfit for human habitation' and among 'fit' dwellings 921,000 lacked one or more of the basic amenities and 1.5 million required repairs costing over £1,000.[76] We do not know how many of these dwellings were inhabited by old people, but it is certain to be a disproportionately high number. An unfit or inadequate house is unlikely to be a warm or comfortable one and our evidence supports this contention (Table 6.2) and yet the findings from the 1976 House Condition Survey, while providing no direct evidence, strongly suggest that a high proportion of the housing stock is inadequately heated, insulated or draught-proofed. The answer to bad housing conditions lies in the continuing application of improvement programmes. As noted earlier, an improved dwelling now has to meet Parker Morris heating standards in order to qualify for improvement grant. Certainly much is to be gained if both owners and housing authorities think increasingly in terms of heating needs when carrying out improvement works.

Housing alternatives

While many old people will wish to stay on in their existing homes, there will be some who will prefer, and will need, to move to better, more appropriate accommodation. What are the options available here? There are, of course, different sorts of problems that call for different kinds of solutions.

Towards the end of the life cycle many people need to move to smaller accommodation. As the Cullingworth Report notes, the elderly 'typically face a problem of too much, rather than too little, space',[77] Our own results show that a significant proportion of pensioners have bedrooms that are not in use and also that they are more likely to have low room temperatures (Table A.11).

Local authorities and housing associations need to become increasingly aware of the deprivations that can be caused by this problem of 'under-occupation' (a term that puts more emphasis on the misuse of housing stock than the problem suffered by the occupiers). A happy home that once bustled with all the activities associated with a growing family can become a bleak and wearisome abode in old age. Some local authorities, now aware of this issue, are willing to buy owner-occupied housing and to rehouse the occupant more appropriately. The subsequent letting of such housing to families offers a double benefit from this policy.

The evidence from our national survey strongly suggests that housing

authorities should become more aware of hypothermia and heating problems when allocating accommodation. Authorities of course face an
enormously difficult task in allocating accommodation in conditions of
scarcity. The most elaborate and sophisticated points scheme will never
be perfect, nor will it satisfy everybody. But we are arguing here for local
authorities to recognize another aspect of housing need which sometimes
(but not always) might be more significant than, say, the lack of a bath or
an inside lavatory.

Turning from allocation to the type of accommodation available, one
can distinguish between ordinary housing and that specially designed with
the needs of the elderly in mind. During the post-war period there has been
a major shortage of small units of accommodation suitable for the old.
Nevertheless, following the heavy emphasis on family housing in the early
post-war period, there has been a substantial redirection of resources
towards one-bedroom housing in recent times. In England and Wales
one-bedroom units represented 30% of all local authority flats built between 1945 and 1960, 46% in 1960 and 62% in 1976. The proportion of
one-bedroom flats built for private owners has also increased during this
period, but in 1976 still represented only 26% of the total.[78] However, as
is recognized in the 1976 consultation paper 'Housing for Old People'
changing household patterns mean that the number of one-bedroom units
provided becomes a less useful indicator of provision for the elderly than it
was in the past.

Ordinary housing, albeit smaller and warmer accommodation, will not
be adequate for the most frail old people. Among the very aged, handicaps
will increase and while a minority will require hospital care or a place in an
old people's home, others will live with friends or relatives. Some, however, require a different sort of housing. They will be those who, though
still independent, require some help with the day-to-day tasks and, possibly, an opportunity to meet other people. For these sheltered housing
will very often be the answer. It is reckoned that in 1965 there were 63,541
elderly people in sheltered housing in England and Wales and it was
estimated that the number would rise to 159,228 by 1971. Efforts are now
being made to obtain more up-to-date information.[79] It is housing of this
kind that will very often be appropriate for those most at risk of becoming
hypothermic.

Conclusions

In this chapter the discussion has ranged widely over a number of matters
that affect the heating needs of the old. All of these subjects, be it standards of insulation, the future of district heating or the pricing policies of

the fuel industries, are (or could be) crucial in their effect on cold conditions. A review of these subjects has really only skimmed the surface of what is a series of related and complex debates. But while their relevance to our concern is obvious, it is also clear that too often the social aspect is lost in a welter of technological and economic analysis. How will new developments affect the ordinary householder? What, in particular, are their advantages and disadvantages for the elderly and the poor? These are the sorts of questions that need to be asked more often in debates about energy and heating policy wherever they occur. In short, Britain needs an energy policy, but it must be one with a human face.

The chapter closed with a discussion about housing needs and policy. While certain specific policies (such as better insulation) should be directed at the 'old and cold' problem, its eradication depends, to a large extent on 'mainstream' policies. Of particular importance is improvement policy. Old people live in poorer housing than others and in these environments it is difficult to keep homes warm. But, while many old people wish to remain in their existing accommodation, others will need to move to smaller dwellings and, for a minority, sheltered housing would be appropriate. Underlining all approaches however is the need for housing authorities to pay special regard to the dangers of hypothermia and the problem of cold conditions.

Summary and Conclusions

Chapter 10
Social Policy and the
Old and Cold

The aim of this final chapter is to summarize the national survey's main findings and to do this in the context of a discussion about the importance of the problem of the old and cold and its implications for policy and administration.

How Great a Problem?

The starting point for our enquiries was that relatively little was known about the size of the problem of hypothermia or the cold elderly. Indeed there were wildly conflicting estimates and many assertions, but few hard facts. We can now summarize our results and discuss them in relation to other findings. Does a clear picture emerge?

From all the reliable evidence now available it is possible to demonstrate that:—

(1) large proportions of the elderly have cold living conditions;
(2) while most of them maintain reasonable inner body temperatures, a significant minority fail to do so and are at risk of developing hypothermia;
(3) of those at risk a small proportion have inner body temperatures below the hypothermic level;
(4) a small (but significant) proportion of elderly hospital admissions are hypothermic; and
(5) an unknown number die from hypothermia in hospitals, in their own homes and elsewhere.

The above conclusions can be discussed with reference to our own and other evidence.

(1) Cold homes

An important finding of the national survey concerned room temperatures. In general many of the elderly live in cold conditions and the majority had living-room and bedroom temperatures below recommended levels. Thus 77% of the sample had morning living-room temperatures at or below 64.4°F (i.e. 0.6°F below the Parker-Morris standard), and 55% were below 60.8°F (16°C) − the minimum temperature specified in the 1963 Offices, Shops and Railway Premises Act. Similarly, bedroom temperatures were very low. Eighty-four per cent of minimum bedroom temperatures were below 60.8°F (16°C) while 33% were below 50°F (10°C). Obviously there is no neat dividing line between cold and warm conditions, and ideas about thermal comfort will vary over time and between people and countries. However, most people would agree that many of Britain's elderly live in cold conditions, and certainly have room temperatures low enough for hypothermia to become a possibility.

(2) The 'at risk'

The second main finding of our survey was that there were some 9.6% of the sample 'at risk' of developing hypothermia (i.e. with morning urine temperatures below 35.5°C). From this figure we can estimate that approximately 700,000 old people were 'at risk' at the time of our survey. These elderly people were 'at risk' because of their small reserves of body heat and because the core to periphery temperature gradient of this group indicated thermoregulatory inadequacy.

A survey undertaken in Camden throws more light on the physiological characteristics of the 'at risk'. This was carried out in 1975−76 on 47 old people who were first surveyed in 1972. It was found in hospital tests that the body core-shell gradients were smaller in 1976, indicating thermoregulatory impairment. The researchers report that their studies 'confirm, both on a cross-sectional and longitudinal basis that there is an age-related decline in autonomic nervous function which leads to impairment of thermoregulatory capacity in a high proportion of old people'.[1]

(3) The number of hypothermics

The third important finding of the national survey was that a small proportion of the sample had hypothermia at the time of the morning interview. In fact there were six subjects with morning urine temperature of 35°C or below and we regarded this as properly constituting hypothermia (see Chapter 4). These six represented 0.58% of the total sample. In fact, due to the rigorous definitions adopted and because it represents a percentage of the whole sample (and not just those whose urine temperatures were successfully measured) this proportion probably represents an underestimate of those with hypothermic temperatures in the morning. On the other hand these were morning temperatures and all were above the hypothermic level the previous evening. As we noted in Chapter 4, this indicates the importance of the circadian rhythm which is probably exacerbated by extremely cold night-time conditions.

In our preliminary report we stated that 'it is most unwise to make firm projections of the incidence of hypothermia for the population as a whole.' This is because the body temperatures fluctuate above and below the arbitrary hypothermic level and because 'the classification of hypothermia would depend on the time of day that the temperature is taken.' We also noted that 'the hypothermia in our two groups of subjects (i.e. 'low' and 'normal') is based on a temperature difference of 0.2°C, which clearly has relatively little biological significance.' One might also add that our findings relate to the period January to March 1972 and we cannot draw firm conclusions about winter periods generally. However, for this discussion it might be helpful to mention the kind of numbers that the figure 0.58 per cent represents. In fact Age Concern had estimated that this proportion represents 44,752 old people aged 65 and over in Great Britain. It is better to talk, more generally, in terms of several tens of thousands with hypothermia at the time of our survey. That probably gives a reasonable idea of the numbers with hypothermia (as defined) but it is a figure that should only be quoted in context and with caution. It demonstrates however the magnitude of the problem.

(4) Hypothermics in hospital

The Royal College of Physicians has carried out two surveys of low body temperature in patients being admitted to hospital. The first was in 1965 and the main findings were discussed in Chapter 1. Briefly, these were that during a three-month period 0.68% of all admissions (and 1.2% of the elderly admitted) were reported as having hypothermia. In 1975 a further enquiry was carried out.[2] This was a pilot study in certain London hospitals belonging to the University College Hospital Group. It found that 3.6% of elderly patients admitted to hospital had hypothermia (i.e. deep body temperature below 35.0°C). Despite it being a milder winter, the authors of the study's report conclude that:

> The findings suggest that the prevalence of hypothermia among the elderly admitted to hospital is even greater than was suggested by the previous Royal College of Physicians' study carried out ten years ago.

There are several possible reasons for this. It might be partly due to the differences between the populations from which the patients were drawn (some of the 1975 sample being found out of doors). It is possible, however, that in 1965 there was an underestimate of the incidence of hypothermia on admission in the old, whereas in 1975 there was a very careful briefing and supervision of all staff. Furthermore the 1965 study was conducted before main hospitals became District General Hospitals and consequently patients most at risk of hypothermia may have been admitted to other hospitals. Bearing in mind these points it would seem that the 1975 figure of 3.6% is a better indicator of the proportion of elderly hospital admissions with hypothermia than the much lower 1965 figure.

The earlier Royal College report estimated that, on the basis of their findings, there were 9,000 hypothermic admissions to all hospitals in the three-month period. However, it is important to bear in mind that this figure was for all age groups.

The authors of the report of the 1975 Pilot Study make no population projections, but clearly, if these findings were representative of hospital admissions generally, the number of elderly patients entering hospitals with hypothermia would be considerable.

It would be helpful to relate the data on hospital admissions to the results of our own survey about the number of elderly people with hypothermia at home. But we are not able to do this. We do not know about the general medical condition of our national sample, nor how many of the hypothermic or 'at risk' group later entered hospital. Nevertheless, it would seem likely that some of those at home with very low body temperatures later entered hospital. We do not know how many, nor do we know the proportion that remain at home with very low body temperatures without hospital care (or any medical attention).

(5) Deaths from hypothermia

Much of the public discussion on hypothermia has centred on the question of death from the condition. Two sets of statistics have dominated the discussion and while they present estimates of deaths which are at opposite extremes from one another, they have in common one factor – their unreliability. On the one hand we often read in the press that 60,000 old people (or even 90,000) will die from hypothermia 'this winter'. On the other hand we are reassuringly told that, in fact, there are only a few deaths from hypothermia each year. What are the origins of these estimates?

At the one extreme is the fact that official statistics suggest that very few deaths from hypothermia occur each year. Table 10.1 gives the estimate of deaths 'attributed solely or mainly to hypothermia'.

These figures are based on death certificates and it is well known – and has been for some time – that these are extremely unreliable on the

Table 10.1

Death Certificates: Deaths 'Attributed Solely or Mainly to Hypothermia' During Six Months, October to March (England and Wales)

1965/66	15
1966/67	8
1967/68	6
1968/69	*
1969/70	*
1970/71	16
1971/72	18
1972/73	10
1973/74	22

* Figures for winter periods not available. Deaths in 18-month period from October 1968 to March 1970 totalled 48.
Source: Hansard, Vol. 888, Col. 509

question of hypothermia. Hypothermia is often difficult to diagnose, particularly where an old person's body is discovered some time after death. The relationship between hypothermia and other illnesses is also complex and while hypothermia may be the prime cause of death, it may be the related illness that is recorded on the death certificate.

The use of death certificates should by now be of only historic interest were it not for the fact that the DHSS continues to use this data in response to questions about hypothermia from concerned Members of Parliament. Their constant use in this way is extremely regrettable. While there is *no* firm evidence on the number of deaths wholly or partly due to hypothermia, our own 1972 survey and the surveys of the Royal College of Physicians, together with the experience of doctors, social workers and others, should long ago have convinced the DHSS that the death-certificate-based hypothermia figures are not merely inaccurate, but totally irrelevant. Their continued use suggests a complacency which fails to match the anxiety of many people about hypothermia.

Statements to the effect that 60,000 old people die from hypothermia every winter derive from the fact that many more people die in the winter months than in the summer. Two points can be made about figures such as these. The first is that they relate to all age groups and not just the elderly. Thus for the period 1961–70 (comparing the periods January–March and October–December of each calendar year with April–September) the average total of winter deaths over and above those occurring in the summer was approximately 65,000. During the very cold winter of 1962/3 94,000 more people died compared to the following summer.[3] This figure gives a good indication of what the effects of a really long and cold winter can be. Another example can be taken from the winter during which our own survey was conducted. Between October 1971 and March 1972 there was a total of approximately 316,100 registered deaths in England and Wales compared to 267,500 during the following summer (i.e. April – September 1972), making an excess of 48,600. However the excess number of winter deaths for people aged 65 years and over was approximately 39,000.[4]

The second point about the figures is that they are obviously not an estimate of deaths from hypothermia. There is a danger that their misuse in the past has led government officials and others to take the problems of the cold elderly less seriously than they should. It is overlooked, to take an extreme example, that there are more deaths from road accidents in the winter than the summer. However, there is a proven relationship between cold weather and death rates. Certain medical conditions are more likely than others to be associated with death in winter and some interesting work has been carried out which relates deaths from some of these to changes in air temperatures. Bull and Morton have found that:—

Changes of temperature of short duration (2 – 10 days) and of longer duration (15 and more days) are associated with inverse changes in death rates in both respiratory infections (pneumonia and bronchitis) and in vascular diseases (myocardial infarction and cerebral vascular accidents). These relationships are less or absent in younger subjects and marked in the elderly.[5]

What can reliably be said about the numbers of the elderly dying of hypothermia? As we note in Chapter 1, in the 1965 Royal College survey 37% of the hypothermic admissions died, but these came from all age groups and in most cases other diseases were present. However there were ten elderly patients in whom hypothermia was the principal diagnosis and five of these died.

The 1975 pilot survey found 22 patients with rectal temperatures below 35°C on admission and of these 10 patients died. Thirteen of the patients were considered to have primary hypothermia, that is 'the principal diagnosis was accidental hypothermia induced by cold exposure in the absence of an obvious clinical cause to account for the lowering of the body temperature'.[6] Five of these patients died. (It is interesting to see that even the results of this one small pilot survey cast serious doubt on the relevance of figures based on death certificates).

We do not know therefore how many of the extra winter deaths are due to, or are associated with, hypothermia. Nevertheless these figures are important in emphasizing the effect of cold weather on morbidity and mortality and, of course, deaths from hypothermia will be crucially affected by the severity of winter. 'Ironically public concern about the plight of the old and cold has developed over a number of winters that have been comparatively mild. Our survey results show that even during such winters many old people have low body temperatures and that many more live in cold conditions. Obviously during a very cold winter the number of deaths from hypothermia will rise, the proportion of the elderly at risk will increase and many more will suffer from miserably cold conditions. How much worse would the problems be when we again have a winter like that of 1962/3 when:

> Just before Christmas, temperatures fell to below freezing point and did not rise much above this again until the end of February. The daily death rate started to rise immediately the cold spell started and remained high for the rest of the winter.[7]

Social Conditions and Low Temperatures

Before drawing together the policy implications of this research, it is useful first to summarize our main findings from the national survey about the association between social and economic circumstances and low body and room temperatures. In Chapter 4 we showed that, contrary to what we expected, there was no statistically significant association between low body and low room temperatures: i.e. people 'at risk' did not necessarily live in the coldest homes. Given this finding, we did not expect to find significant associations between low body temperatures and those socio-economic factors that directly bear on the level of room temperatures. But why do a minority of the elderly fail to maintain an adequate deep body temperature (while many others, many of them in cold conditions, preserve core temperature homeostasis)?

Age would appear to be an important factor: in general the very aged are more at risk than younger pensioners. But this point, while important, should not be exaggerated, for many younger pensioners are also at risk.

Poverty was not directly related to low core temperature, but the receipt of supplementary benefit was. This was an interesting finding and we suggested that the receipt of benefits might be an indicator of multiple deprivation which has a causal relation to low body temperature. The relationship between age, the receipt of supplementary benefits and low core temperatures was explored. We found that, in fact, it was very aged supplementary pensioners who were most vulnerable. This is probably due to the effects of a declining physiology (perhaps exacerbated by illness) combined with the most deprived social conditions.

Two factors that might reasonably be expected to have an immediate influence on body temperatures were found to be significantly associated with the 'at risk' group. One was body weight (as assessed by our nurse-interviewers) and we found that the underweight subjects were more likely to be at risk. The other was electric blankets and we found that those using them were less likely to be at risk than those using hot-water bottles or relying on extra blankets during the winter.

In Chapter 5 we analysed the old people's feelings about the cold, their 'comfort votes', their preferences for warmth and their perceptions of the cold. We concluded that, in general, people at risk are more likely than others to report they often feel cold indoors, have cold hands and prefer more warmth. Similarly those living in the coldest rooms are generally more likely to be cold and want greater warmth. However, we also found that large proportions of the at risk and of those in the coldest housing reported that they did *not* often feel cold indoors, that their hands did *not* get cold, that they would *not* prefer to be warmer, and so on. Such results need to be interpreted cautiously. In some cases they might reflect not so much a person's failure to feel the cold, but rather an unwillingness to report, or admit to, feeling cold and prefering to be warmer. This might be due to pride, independence, or a general reluctance to complain. In other cases the explanation might be the old person's failure to feel cold as body temperature falls during cold periods. It is also likely that the old are more used to, and tolerant of, the cold than younger groups who expect, and are used to, higher standards. But whatever the reasons for our results, they offer no encouragement to medical practitioners and social service staff concerned with the prevention and identification of hypothermia.

In Chapter 6 we turned our attention to cold homes, that is to low room temperatures rather than low body temperatures. The findings show that there are no short-cuts to identifying those in the coldest homes in terms of sex, marital status, household composition or age. Regarding housing, council tenants are more likely to have warmer bedrooms, while dwellings lacking basic amenities have colder bedrooms. Purpose-built flats were warmer than other house types, and elderly people with one or more bedrooms seldom in use had colder homes.

Less than one quarter of the sample had central heating. But those with it used central heating regularly and had significantly warmer homes than others. We found that only one in ten of the elderly heated their bedrooms 'all night' and almost a half did not heat them at all.

The effect of financial hardship on heating is difficult to assess because many other factors are influential. It is also important to remember that most of the elderly are poor, relative to the rest of the population. As expected most of the elderly found heating expensive and cost was the major reason why those wanting more heat in the house did not have it. The 'at risk' and those in the coldest rooms were neither more nor less likely than others to be receiving social service callers or be in contact with their doctors. Nevertheless the finding that one quarter of the at risk had not seen a doctor for more than a year is disturbing.

Identifying those at risk

Our research offers no easy ways of identifying those 'at risk' or the elderly living in the coldest homes. Indeed a major finding of this research is that these groups are to be found throughout the whole of the elderly population, despite differences of income, household composition, housing tenure, physical mobility and so on. Also, we have already noted that many of those 'at risk' and most in need of help are unlikely to report that they feel cold and require warmer conditions.

Thus one cannot rely on old people themselves coming forward for help. However, while it is not possible to point to particular groups that contain all or the vast majority of the 'at risk' and cold elderly, certain factors are important and can be used as guidelines by those concerned with identification and prevention.

As the discussion in Chapter 5 showed, advancing age and the receipt of supplementary benefits are significantly associated with being at risk. Where these two factors are found together, vulnerability is considerably increased. Thus, at one extreme, 26% of supplementary benefit recipients aged 85 and over were at risk – almost four times as many as all pensioners not receiving benefit. We also found that the use of electric blankets seemed to reduce the risk of developing hypothermia. Similarly body weight appears to be an important factor. Thus one can build up a profile of those likely to be physically vulnerable to the cold. But these factors are just guidelines and many of those at risk do not fall into these categories – half of the 'low' temperature group were in fact not receiving supplementary benefit for example.

The particular vulnerability of those living alone – and especially the socially isolated – must be recognized. The aged person living alone – particularly if he or she does not keep regularly in touch with people – will face particular dangers if body temperature starts to fall.

The problem of identifying and then helping those at risk is part of the wider problem of meeting the needs of the aged whether they relate to cold housing or to such problems as physical handicap, poor nutrition and loneliness. However, it is important that when social services departments or other agencies carry out research on local needs or consider the drawing up of 'risk' registers, the dangers from the cold should be a prime consideration. How can social and health services identify those at risk? In fact a considerable proportion of the elderly are already regularly visited by staff from one part or another of the 'welfare state'. Although only 15% of the sample were visited by 'domiciliary callers' – e.g. home helps, health visitors etc. – who might be expected to be most alert to the danger of low body temperatures – as many as 37% received a caller from social service, health, housing or voluntary bodies. By far the most important category was the 'rent man' who called on 23% of our sample.

There is therefore a solid foundation on which to launch an effective preventive campaign to tackle problems such as the 'old and cold'. The Department of Health's 'Good Neighbour Scheme', if properly developed, could play a major part in such a service. Meanwhile – as a matter of urgency – there is a need to ensure that all callers are made aware of the problem of hypothermia, its danger signals and where specialised help can be sought. It is also important to involve others who provide services for the elderly, such as postmen and milkmen, in the campaign against hypothermia. It is therefore important that trade unions should be involved in the planning of any such campaign.

While great opportunities exist, there is a possibility that without effective planning, problems could become more acute in the future for the isolated and at risk. There is an increasing tendency for social security and housing staff to make fewer personal contacts with claimants and tenants. In the case of supplementary benefits home visiting has declined and a system of postal reviews has been developed. The effect is that years may pass before a supplementary benefits officer has any need to visit a supplementary pensioner. Similarly, the number of door-to-door rent collections has declined, replaced by the giro or the payment of rents at local offices. These changes, made for the benefit of the service provider and not the service receiver, can have serious human consequences to which bureaucracies need to address themselves.

Finally, it is important to emphasise the need for using low reading clinical thermometers in the identification and diagnosis of hypothermia. An ordinary thermometer fails to record this condition and yet many doctors still only use this type. It is essential that doctors, nurses and health visitors use low reading thermometers particularly when caring for groups susceptible to hypothermia, such as the old and new-born babies.

Social policy: conclusions and recommendations

The identification of those suffering from low body or room temperatures is the obvious first step, but what further action should be taken to tackle these problems? In Chapters 7, 8 and 9 we looked at several areas of policy – social security, heating, housing and personal social services – and the way in which benefits and services in these fields do or could make an impact on the problem of the old and the cold. We can now draw together some of the conclusions of our study and present some specific recommendations that emerge from our work, as well as some more general conclusions.

Social Security

In Chapter 7 we focused on the supplementary benefits system and in particular on the award of discretionary additions. Our own survey demonstrated that benefit recipients are often ignorant about the existence of weekly heating additions and systems of this kind are inevitably complex and hard to understand. Not surprisingly it is officially estimated that one in three of those eligible for this extra cash help do not in fact receive it.

There is now more known about heating additions than at the time of our survey. Many more supplementary pensioners now receive them. The DHSS has recently given them some publicity, but much more should be done. Action should include not only the distribution of leaflets for social service and voluntary workers and the elderly themselves (and other benefit recipients) but also newspaper, radio and television advertising. Such advertising presents problems for social security officers and runs the risk of raising hopes that cannot be met. Nevertheless if it enabled more old people to receive extra cash help towards their heating costs, such advertising would be well worthwhile.

As we argued in Chapter 7 reliance on a system of heating additions presents no real solution to meeting heating needs. The possibility of paying full heating costs should be seriously explored by the DHSS. But even such a radical proposal is not ideal. It offers no help to those of the elderly – some 600,000 pensioners – who do not receive supplementary pensions despite their being eligible for them, nor to many more of the elderly who, although ineligible for benefit, are not in fact much better off than those receiving it. A means-tested approach to income support in old age offers no hope of eradicating poverty as a cause of cold conditions.

Two important points can be made about lump sum exceptional needs payments (ENPs). Unlike extra weekly additions, the award of an ENP for heating equipment, say, offers a means of tackling the problem of inadequate warmth at its root. One must not overstate this argument. The SBC is *not* a housing authority, nor should it or could it enter into the business of large-scale housing improvement. However the SBC should review its policy towards the award of ENPs to see what scope exists to tackle some of the heating and insulating problems faced by its clients.

The second point about ENPs concerns the provision of electric blankets. The current policy of the Commission is that ENPs should not be awarded for electric blankets. The SBC's problems must be acknowledged here. Where do its responsibilities end and those of other agencies start? And should it provide its claimants with goods or services which those ineligible for benefit might not be able to afford? Nevertheless, having recognized these problems, one can make a strong case for a change in the Commissions's policy. One of the more specific results from the national survey strongly suggests that the use of electric blankets is an effective preventive measure in the fight against hypothermia. It is ironic that ENPs are awarded for hot-water bottles which those at risk use more than those with normal temperatures, but not for the one night-time safeguard that our results suggest is relatively effective.

The only substantial argument against providing electric blankets concerns safety. The number of deaths involving electric blankets is relatively small, but most of the deaths occur in the elderly population. Safety is then an important issue, but what is required is a positive approach towards it. Surely it would be more responsible for the DHSS to advise on the safest blankets available (and to encourage development of even safer ones) than to discourage their use when they can effectively prevent low body temperatures? There is, after all, an element of danger about all artificial methods of keeping warm and yet no one would seriously suggest proscribing all forms of heating. And of course, although there is no evidence, it is arguable that the use of electric blankets by those 'at risk' could prevent far more deaths than might be caused by the occasional misuse of such blankets.

Personal social services

From our survey of social service authorities in Greater London (the results of which were reported in Chapter 8) the following conclusions emerged.

It was clear that many local authority social services departments defined the problem too narrowly – as a specific problem of hypothermia, a medical condition. Rather, we argued, the problem should be seen in more general terms. Departments should be concerned with the miserably cold conditions in which millions of elderly people live.

Local authorities should also be more aware of the potential and strength of existing legislation. Much more extensive and imaginative use could be made of the powers which already exist. Local authorities should make full use of the services, aids and appliances that can most effectively contribute to an attack on the problems of the old and the cold.

Heating and Housing

Ensuring that all old people have adequately heated homes involves a number of issues in the fields of housing, heating, energy and other policy areas. Some of these issues are exceedingly complex, such as the future development of district heating, and involve the making of fundamental decisions which will affect future generations. However, from the analysis presented in Chapter 9, several points emerge. The first point concerns home insulation. While its advantages have become more and more recognized in recent years, it is likely that those most in need will stand the least chance of having their homes insulated. It is important therefore that the government, in association with the local authorities, trade unions and voluntary bodies, should launch a national programme to ensure that the elderly in need have their homes adequately insulated. By using the skills of unemployed construction workers and the labour of the unemployed young, and in view of the consequent energy savings, this policy offers both economic and social advantages.

The second point concerns the pricing policies in the fuel industries. It is clear that very often those most in need, including many of the elderly, pay more for the fuel they consume than others. It is important that government, and the fuel industries themselves, review their policies to ensure that any discrimination that exists should be in favour of, and not against, the poorest consumers. Finally we would place emphasis on the need for housing authorities to allow fully for the dangers of hypothermia and cold conditions in the allocation of housing. This means, among other things, recognizing that too much space may lead to cold conditions.

Responsibility and Coordination

We have been able to make some recommendations in certain specific fields of social policy. However, the problems of the old and cold do not fall into neat social policy areas; they are not all adequately catered for by the existing division of social services. Indeed the 'old and cold' problem is a major example of how, despite a relatively sophisticated range of social services and benefits, gaps in provision occur and overlaps are found producing confusions as to who exactly is responsible for what.

A number of different social service agencies and public bodies have responsibilities which are directly relevant to the heating needs of the elderly. It may be that the local authority housing department meets the need. At best an old person might live in purpose-built accommodation with effective central heating. At worst the elderly council tenant might be living in cold and draughty housing with ineffective heating appliances. In practice the SBC also has an important role. It not only pays out large numbers of heating additions, but it can also make lump sum payments for heating appliances. Local authority social service departments are also able to distribute heating appliances and the local electricity and gas boards have responsibilities that they should not ignore. It all adds up to an extremely confusing picture not only for the elderly themselves, but also for the various agencies, voluntary bodies and concerned neighbours, friends and relations.

What needs to be done?

There is a need for rationalization and clarification of responsibilities at both local and national levels. At local level one agency should take the lead in mobilizing help to tackle heating problems. Are the problems faced by one old lady best tackled by (a) seeking local authority housing (with central heating)?; (b) easing anxiety about cost (by applying for a heating addition, if the old person receives supplementary benefit)?; (c) providing roof insulation (by means, perhaps, of an improvement grant) and organizing the labour (from a voluntary body) to lay it down?; (d) negotiating with the gas or electricity board (if there is a debt)?; (e) the wearing of warmer clothing, which might be purchased with the help of an ENP or obtained from the social services department?; or (f) applying for a heating appliance or an electric blanket from the social services department? There are a range of possibilities and while sometimes the old person, or a friend or relation, will know how to seek the right help, in many other cases they will not.

The appropriate agency to carry out this responsibility is, we believe, the local authority social services department. Apart from taking the lead in identifying the 'at risk' their role should be to (1) act as an initial channel of communication, receiving and processing requests for information and help; (2) coordinate provision from different social service agencies; (3) mobilize and coordinate community and voluntary organizations.

At the national level a more ambitious task needs to be undertaken. Government reponses to the 'old and cold' problem to date have been piecemeal and have seriously failed to match the seriousness of the situation. Different departments: – Energy, Environment and Health and Social Security – have looked at aspects of their own policies and services, but central government has not carried out a comprehensive examination of the 'old and cold' problem to assess what corporate response can be made. This failure is an example of a broader problem which has been recognized by the Central Policy Review Staff. In their report *A Joint Framework for Social Policies* the CPRS highlighted the need for 'improved coordination between services as they affect the individual' and 'better analysis of, and policy prescriptions for, complex problems – especially when they are the concern of more than one department.'[8]

What is required is for central government to look comprehensively at the 'old and cold' problem with a view to developing a programme that would ensure that all old people have warm homes, regardless of their domestic or financial circumstances.

Hypothermia and Social Policy

The above discussion presents the major recommendations that emerged from our review of different policy areas. They all, in different ways, entail *specific* attacks on the problem of low body and environmental temperatures – by using electric blankets, providing heating additions, insulating housing, etc. However, while great importance should be attached to such measures – and while some could make a major impact – the best hope of tackling the adverse effect of low temperatures lies in a more general approach.

To state one of our major findings once more, while certain groups of the old are more 'at risk' than others, those with low body and room temperatures are to be found throughout the elderly population. The policy implication of this is that the successful attack on cold conditions cannot come through a selective strategy. It is not simply a question of more and more heating additions (for non-recipients of supplementary benefits are not eligible for these) nor is it just a question of extra vigilant (and specially trained) welfare staff (for the vast majority of the at risk will never receive a call from them). Rather a universal approach is necessary. And while this involves a number of policy areas, emphasis should be placed on two of them: housing and social security.

In housing there is tremendous unmet demand among the elderly for smaller units of accommodation and for housing specially built for their needs. Sheltered housing is particularly important. However, new construction makes a slow impression on general housing conditions and therefore improvement policy is all-important. This can make a direct impact on cold conditions (through the provision of heating systems and insulation) but at least as important is the general raising of standards that leads to better amenities, damp-free accommodation and greater comfort.

Social security is equally important. Although incomes vary a good deal among the elderly, there is no doubt that in general terms the elderly are relatively poor compared to the rest of the population. A selected means-tested approach offers no way forward. The solution can only come through a significant increase in the level of pensions. Like the housing proposals, this is a costly policy approach. But this book's analysis shows that hypothermia cannot be tackled inexpensively.

The analysis of the problem of the 'old and cold' presented in this book and the review of the existing range of services and policies points to a four-fold strategy. The first part concerns identification. At the extreme, cold conditions can result in lonely tragedy – death from hypothermia, unsuspected and undetected by relatives, neighbours or the apparatus of the welfare state. There is a need to develop a preventive campaign which would involve not only 'welfare' staff but also relations, neighbours and others who regularly call on the old. Secondly there are a number of fairly immediate or short-term measures that should be undertaken, which would have a direct impact on cold conditions. These include wider and more determined publicity for supplementary benefit heating additions and the launching of a programme to bring the benefits of home insulation to the old. Thirdly there is a need for co-ordination at both local and national levels to ensure that gaps in provision do not occur and to make a comprehensive approach possible. Finally, and most importantly, it is necessary to recognize that it is only through the development of main-stream policies for the elderly that problems associated with the cold can be eradicated. These cover a range of services and issues, but the most important concern housing and social security.

It cannot be assumed that the problems discussed in this book have lessened in any way since the time of our survey, nor that they will automatically be overcome in the future. In fact there are grounds for thinking the opposite. The numbers of very aged – those in their late seventies, eighties, nineties and older – have increased and will increase at a faster rate than those of younger pensioners. The very pensioners who are most at risk are therefore becoming more numerous. Also, increasing heating costs have meant that many more pensioners are not able to keep adequately warm in the winter. Finally, anxiety about hypothermia has developed over a number of winters that have been relatively mild. Sooner or later a very severe winter will occur again. How will our old people fare when this happens? Will the widespread anxiety that exists about hypothermia, the interest of the mass media, the campaigns of pressure groups and the concern of government be translated into positive action to ensure that Britain becomes a society where it is no longer possible to be both old and cold?

References

Chapter 1: Hypothermia

1 *Lancet,* 19 March 1955.
2 'Neonatal Cold Injury due to Accidental Exposure to Cold', *Lancet,* 2 February 1957.
3 'Accidental Hypothermia', *Lancet,* 1958, Vol. 1, p. 556.
4 'Accidental Hypothermia: A Common Condition with a Pathognomonic Electro-Cardiogram', *Lancet,* 1958, Vol. 2, p. 492.
5 G. S. Crockett, *British Medical Journal,* 1964, Vol. 1, p. 61.
   H. Duguid, R. G. Simpson, J. M. Stowers, 'Accidental Hypothermia', *Lancet,* 1961, Vol. 2, p. 1213.
   M. W. McNicol, R. Smith, 'Accidental Hypothermia', *British Medical Journal,* 1964, Vol. 1, pp. 19–21.
   J. W. Paulley *et al., British Medical Journal,* 1964, Vol. 1, p. 428.
   L. F. Prescott, M. C. Peard, I. R. Wallace, *British Medical Journal,* 1962, Vol. 2, p. 1367.
   A. J. Rosin, A. N. Exton-Smith, 'Clinical Features of Accidental Hypothermia, with some observations on Thyroid Function', *British Medical Journal,* 4 January 1964.
   J. A. P. Trafford, A. Hopkins, *British Medical Journal,* 1963, **1,** 400.
6 'The Problem of Hypothermia in the Elderly', *The Practitioner,* December 1964, Vol. 193.
7 'Accidental Hypothermia in the Elderly', *British Medical Journal,* 1964, Vol. 2, p. 1255.
8 *Gerontologia Clinica,* 1968, **10,** 281–7.
9 Society of Medical Officers of Health, *Public Health,* 1968, Vol. 82, No. 5.
10 *Public Health,* 1969, Vol. 83, No. 5.
11 Royal College of Physicians, *Report of the Committee on Accidental Hypothermia,* 1966.
12 'The Problem of Hypothermia in the Elderly', op. cit.
13 L. F. Howitt, 'Death in Scotland from Malnutrition and/or Hypothermia, 1968', Scottish Home and Health Department, *Health Bulletin,* January 1971, Vol. 29, No. 1.
14 Jill Harling and Stephen Gullick, *A Study of Living Conditions among the Aged in Birmingham,* carried out by students of Birmingham University for the Wallace Lawler Friendship Fund, July 1969.
15 *Old and Cold in Islington . . . A Question of Survival,* survey carried

out by Islington Task Force and published by them in conjunction with Islington Poverty Action Group and Islington Consumers' Group. *See also* Lilian Fleet, *Left in the Cold,* Task Force (undated).

16 R. H. Fox, 'Physiological Aspects, Results of National and Camden Surveys', *Symposium on Hypothermia, Heating and the Elderly,* Centre for Environmental Studies, January 1975, p. 2.

17 ibid., p. 2.

18 ibid., p. 3.

19 'Accidental Hypothermia in the Elderly', op. cit.

20 *See* L. F. Howitt, op. cit.

21 Michael F. Green, *Hypothermia,* Appendix 3, 'Paying for Fuel', National Consumer Council. HMSO, 1976, p. 132. Green also makes the point that 'In some circumstances hypothermia may be untreatable, as it is a reflection of the inexorable decline in body functions in someone who is dying.'

22 ibid., p. 29.

23 'Accidental Hypothermia in the Elderly', op. cit., p. 1255.

24 Royal College of Physicians, op. cit., p. 4.

25 ibid., table 3 and p. 9.

26 'Accidental Hypothermia in the Elderly', op. cit., p. 1256.

27 ibid., p. 1256.

Chapter 2: The Social Circumstances of Britain's Elderly

1 R. M. Titmuss, *Essays on the Welfare State,* George Allen & Unwin, 1963, p. 56.

2 *Social Trends,* No 7, 1976, HMSO, 1976 Table 1.

3 Department of Health and Social Security Conference on the Elderly, 26 July 1977. *Background Paper,* para 3.

4 *Social Trends,* No 5, 1974, HMSO 1974, Table 28.

5 *Social Trends,* No 7, 1976, HMSO 1976, Table 2.18.

6 *Census 1971. Great Britain.* Age, Marital Condition and General Tables, HMSO, 1974.

7 The figures for 1951 and 1961 are quoted in Jeremy Tunstall, *Old and Alone,* Routledge & Kegan Paul, 1966, p. 46. The 1971 figure is from Office of Population Censuses and Surveys, *Census 1971, Great Britain,* Persons of Pensionable Age, HMSO 1974, Table 2.

8 *General Household Survey,* reports, for 1972, 1973 and 1974, HMSO.

9 *General Household Survey,* report for 1973, Table 1.3.

10 *General Household Survey, Introductory Report,* HMSO, 1973, p. 55.

11 A. N. Exton-Smith, 'Accidental Hypothermia', *British Medical Journal,* 22 December 1973, p. 727.

12 Shanas, Townsend *et al., Old People in Three Industrial Societies,* Routledge & Kegan Paul, 1968. J. Tunstall, op. cit.

13 Shanas, Townsend *et al.,* op. cit., p. 262.

14 ibid., p. 264.

15   *See* Shanas, Townsend *et al,* op. cit. Table II—10.

16   A. N. Exton-Smith, 'Medical Aspects of Hypothermia', *Symposium on Hypothermia, Heating and the Elderly,* Centre for Environmental Studies, 14 January 1975, p. 4.

17   *See* the evidence presented by Shanas, Townsend *et al.,* op. cit., p. 215 and Table VII—26.

18   The General Household Survey estimate of households for 1971 was 30.7% in Great Britain; the Department of Environment estimate for Great Britain was 35.7% for the same year; and the National House Condition Survey figure was 31.4% (for England and Wales). *See* Table 5.3, *General Household Survey 1971, Introductory Report.*

19   Table 2.16, *General Household Survey 1973,* HMSO, 1976. For further evidence *see Census 1971. Great Britain.* Persons of Pensionable Age, HMSO, 1974.

20   Defined by Section 4 of the 1957 Housing Act.

21   That is: internal WC; fixed bath; wash basin; and hot and cold water at 3 points.

22   There is no direct evidence for this, but the elderly generally live in accommodation that is older than that occupied by the rest of the community (Table 2.2 of this chapter); the 1973 General Household Survey shows that the elderly owner-occupier is more likely to own his house outright (Table 2.1 of this 1973 Survey); and that such dwellings are older (Table 2.3) and more likely to lack amenities than houses still being bought with the aid of a mortgage (Table 2.5).

23   *General Household Survey 1973.* Table 2.5(c). The Report distinguishes between 'night storage heaters only' and 'other central heating'. The figures noted in the text include both types. Altogether 9% of all households had night storage heaters only and 30% 'other central heating only'.

24   *General Household Survey 1973.* Table 2.12. For definition of the 'bedroom standard' *see General Household Survey, Introductory Report* op. cit., p. 13.

25   There is no current information available about the precise financial circumstances of elderly people. However a general indication of the income levels of the elderly compared to the rest of the population is provided by the 1972 General Household Survey. For one-person households the median gross weekly income for those aged 16—59 was contained in the range £20—25, while for those aged 60 or over it was in the range £7.50—£10. For two-person households aged 16—59 the relevant income range was £25—30 and for two-person households aged 60+ where one or both were aged 60+ it was £12.50—£15. Although these figures give only a very general guide (the 60+ group contain, for example, elderly persons who are still working) they do show the relative poverty of the elderly.

26   Ministry of Pensions and National Insurance, *Report of an Inquiry by the Ministry of Pensions and National Insurance with the co-operation of the National Assistance Board,* HMSO 1966.

27   Shanas, Townsend *et al.,* op. cit., p. 414.

28   ibid, Table XII—5.

29   *Social Trends,* No 7, 1976, HMSO, 1976, Table 5.32.

30 Supplementary Benefits Commission, *Annual Report, 1976,* Cmnd 6910, September 1977, Table 2.1 and para. 2.9.
31 Supplementary Benefits Commission, *Annual Report 1975* Cmnd 6615, September 1976, para 5.3.
32 Ministry of Pensions & National Insurance, *Financial and Other Circumstances of Retirement Pensioners,* HMSO, 1966.
33 Cmnd. 6615, op. cit., para 2.6. *See also,* Frank Field, 'Unclaimed Benefits', *New Society,* 21 July 1977; National Consumer Council, *Means Tested Benefits,* Discussion Paper, National Consumer Council, 1976; and Ruth Lister, *Take-Up of Means-Tested Benefits,* Child Poverty Action Group, 1974.

Chapter 3: Scientific Methods and Survey Techniques

1 R. H. Fox, 'Physiological Aspects. Results of National and Camden Surveys', op. cit., p. 8.
2 ibid., p. 9.
3 R. H. Fox, R. MacGibbon, Louise Davies, Patricia M. Woodward, 'Problems of the Old and Cold', *British Medical Journal,* 6 January 1973.
4 Shanas, Townsend *et. al.,* op. cit.
5 A. J. Watts, 'Hypothermia in the Aged: a study of the role of cold-sensitivity', *Environmental Research,* 1972, Vol. 5, p. 119.

Chapter 4: Body and Environmental Temperatures

1 R. H. Fox *et. al.,* 'Body Temperatures in the Elderly', *British Medical Journal,* 27 January 1973, Vol. 1, p. 204.
2 R. H. Fox, Patricia M. Woodward, A. J. Fry, J. C. Collins and I. C. MacDonald, 'Diagnosis of Accidental Hypothermia of the Elderly', *Lancet,* 1971, Vol. 1, p. 424.
3 R. H. Fox *et. al.,* 'Body Temperatures in the Elderly', op. cit., p. 205.
4 ibid., p. 204.
5 ibid., p. 203.
6 ibid., p. 202.

Chapter 5: 'At Risk'

1 *Hypothermia,* Appendix 3, 'Paying for Fuel', National Consumer Council, HMSO, 1976, pp. 128–9.
2 'Accidental Hypothermia in the Elderly', *British Medical Journal,* 14 November 1964.

Chapter 6: Cold Homes and Social Conditions

1 Department of the Environment, *Housing and Construction Statistics*, 1, HMSO, 1972, Table 23(c).
2 Supplementary Benefits Commission, *Annual Report 1976*, op. cit., para 12.3.

Chapter 7: Social Security

1 Supplementary Benefits Commission, *Annual Report* HMSO, *1976*, Cmnd. 6910, September 1977, Table 2.1.
For a brief description of the operation of the supplementary benefits system *see* the *Annual Reports* of the Supplementary Benefits Commission, HMSO (published separately since 1975); *see* also Department of Health and Social Security, Supplementary Benefits Commission, *Supplementary Benefits Handbook*, HMSO, various editions; Tony Lynes, *Penguin Guide to Supplementary Benefits*, Penguin 1972; and Ruth Lister, *Supplementary Benefit Rights*, Arrow, 1974.
2 Department of Health and Social Security, Supplementary Benefits Commission, *Supplementary Benefits Handbook*, HMSO, November 1972 edition, para. 37.
3 ibid., para. 37.
4 Supplementary Benefits Commission, *Annual Report*, 1975, op. cit., para. 3.4.
5 *See* the *Report of the National Assistance Board*, HMSO, 1965, Cmnd. 3042, July 1966.
6 *Supplementary Benefits Handbook*, op. cit., para. 58.
7 Ministry of Pensions and National Insurance, *Financial and other Circumstances of Retirement Pensioners*, HMSO, 1966.
8 *See* Chapters 3 and 4 of A. B. Atkinson's *Poverty in Britain and the Reform of Social Security*, Cambridge University Press, 1969; and Tony Lynes, op. cit.
9 *Supplementary Benefits Handbook*, November 1972, op. cit., para. 64.
10 The SBC recognized the problem: '... recipients of supplementary benefit and their advisers will sometimes be unsure whether an additional payment can be made to meet a special expense, ... or whether it would be regarded as covered by the long term addition.' *Supplementary Benefits Handbook*, op. cit., para. 67.
11 Lynes, op, cit., p. 83.
12 The account of this case is based on the Law Report in *The Times*, 21 February 1973.
13 *See* Heating Action Group, *A Guide to Allowances for Families and Old People*, undated, p. 9.
14 The other exceptions were where the ECA is to meet the requirements of a child and where it is to make up the difference between the rent addition paid to a non-householder and his actual rent.

15 *Report of the National Assistance Board for the year ending 31 December 1965*, Cmnd. 3042, HMSO, 1966, p. 20.
16 *SBC Annual Report*, 1975, op. cit., para. 3.5.
17 ibid., para. 3.7.
18 *SBC Annual Report*, 1976, op. cit., Table 12.3. A footnote to this table explains that the 1971 figures are for the number of 'reckonable expenses' allowed rather than the actual number of additions since at that time special needs for heating were still offset against the margin for special needs in the long-term scales.
19 ibid., para. 12.9.
20 A distinction between 'officer discretion' and 'agency discretion' has been made by David Bull in 'Dear David Donnison: The Commission's discretion', *Social Work Today*, Vol. 6, No. 14, 1975.
21 'Keeping Warm in Winter', DHSS, September 1972. This states: 'To keep old people warm in winter the living-room temperature should be about 70°F when the temperature outside is 30°F. Bathrooms and bedrooms should be kept at the same temperature if possible but in any event should be kept warm.'
22 'Dear David Bull, Frank Field, Michael Hill and Ruth Lister', *Social Work Today*, Vol. 6, No. 20, 1976.
23 'Welfare "Rights", Law and Discretion', *Political Quarterly*, Vol. 42, No. 2, 1971, p. 127.
24 ibid., p. 126.
25 *Claimant or Client?* George Allen & Unwin, 1973, pp. 25–6; The distinction between 'creative' and 'proportional' justice has been made by P. Tillich in *Love, Power and Justice*, Oxford University Press, 1960.
26 'Welfare "Rights", Law and Discretion', op. cit.; and David Bull, op. cit.
27 R. Titmuss, op. cit., pp. 125–6.
28 Michael J. Hill, 'The Excercise of Discretion in the National Assistance Board', *Public Administration*, Spring 1969.
29 ibid., p. 81.
30 *SBC Annual Report*, 1975, op. cit., para. 2.19.
31 ibid., para. 2.20.
32 ibid., para. 2.18.
33 'Dear David Bull . . .', op. cit., p. 623.
34 op. cit., p. 125.
35 A precedent of sorts exists in the extra sum (currently 25p) payable in the long-term rate where the claimant or a dependent is aged 80 or over.
36 *SBC Annual Report*, 1976, op. cit., paras. 12.10 and 12.11.
37 ibid., para. 7.23.
38 'Exceptional needs payments', Supplementary Benefits Administration Paper No. 4, DHSS, SBC, HMSO, 1973.
39 *SBC Annual Report*, 1976, op. cit., Table 7.4.
40 ibid., para. 1.37.
41 *SBC Annual Report*, 1975, op. cit., para. 2.35.
42 *SBC Annual Report*, 1976, op. cit., para. 2.12.
43 R. Titmuss, op. cit., p. 131.

44 *Social Trends*, No. 7, HMSO, 1976. Table 5.32.
45 *'Proposals for a Tax-Credit System'*, Cmnd. 5116, HMSO October 1977, para. 110.
46 Cmnd. 5713, HMSO September 1974.
47 Hansard, 29 November 1974, Written Answer, Cols. 289-290.

Chapter 8: Personal Social Services

1   Section 21(i).
2   The overlap between the elderly and physically handicapped groups is often exaggerated. As Marjorie Bucke points out ('Promoting the Welfare of Old People', *The Year Book of Social Policy*, 1971, ed. K. Jones): 'The total population over the age of sixty-five is about seven million, and the number 'handicapped and impaired' and living in their own home is estimated at 1,787,240 – approximately one quarter of the total.'
3   National Assistance Act, Section 31(i).
4   Statutory Instruments, 1971, No. 423 (C.11), 16 March 1971.
5   'Welfare of the Elderly'. Implementation of Section 45 of the Health Services and Public Health Act, 1968, para. 2.
6   ibid., para. 4.
7   ibid., para. 6.
8   ibid., para. 7.
9   loc. cit.
10 ibid., para. 4f.
11 DHSS Circular 12/70. The Chronically Sick and Disabled Persons Act 1970, para. 5.
12 loc. cit.
13 'Social Administration Digest', *Journal of Social Policy*, Vol. 1, Part 3, July 1972, para. 6.7.
14 DHSS Circular 33/72; DOE Circular 88/72, 25 August 1972.
15 ibid., para. 1.
16 ibid., para 2.
17 loc. cit.
18 ibid., para. 3.
19 ibid., para. 5.
20 Anthony Hall and Malcolm Wicks, 'Winning the Cold War for Old People', *Community Care*, 11 June 1975.
21 'Winter Campaign to Save the Elderly at Risk', *Community Care*, 10 December 1975.
22 Social Services Research, London Borough of Hillingdon, 'Heating and the Elderly: A review of research and long-term policy', February 1974.

Chapter 9: Housing and Heating

1   *Heating and Ventilation of Dwellings* (The Egerton Report). By the Heating and Ventilation Reconstruction Committee of the Building Research Branch of the Department of Scientific and Industrial

Research, Ministry of Works, Post-War Building Studies No. 19. HMSO, 1945.
2 ibid., para. 1.1.1.
3 ibid., para. 2.1.1.
4 ibid., para. 2.1.5.1. For the committee's definition of 'equivalent temperature' *see* para. 2.1.3. of the report.
5 ibid., para. 2.1.6.
6 'Heating of Dwellings Inquiry.' A survey of 5,268 Working Class Households, made in February and March 1942 for the Department of Scientific and Industrial Research Wartime Social Survey. Also reported in Appendix 1 of the Egerton Report, op. cit.
7 ibid., papers 12 and 14.
8 Leslie T. Wilkins, *Domestic utilisation of Heating Appliances and Expenditure on Fuels in 1948/49*. The Social Survey, Central Office of Information, 1951.
9 ibid., Table A/2.
10 ibid., p. 14.
11 P. G. Gray, *The Use of Heating Appliances and the Expenditure on Fuel by Urban Households Living in Dwellings of medium and low rateable values*. An inquiry made for the Building Research Station in 1952. The Social Survey, Central Office of Information, 1954.
12 ibid., p. 10. *See also* P. G. Gray, *Domestic Heating*. An inquiry made for the Building Research Station in 1955. The Social Survey, Central Office of Information.
13 Ministry of Housing and Local Government, *Homes for today and tomorrow*, HMSO, 1961.
14 ibid., para. 65. The high standards recommended by the Institution of Heating and Ventilating Engineers (I.H.V.E.) can also be noted. Central heating capable of reaching a minimum of 21°C in the living and dining room is recommended. *See* Study Group on Domestic Engineering, *Domestic Engineering Services*, I.H.V.E. 1974.
15 ibid., para. 69.
16 'Housing Standards and Costs. Accommodation Specially Designed for Old People', 24 October 1969, Circular 82/69. *See* section F on space heating.
17 Housing Development Notes, 4. 'Thermal Insulation in Housing.' 1. 'The Case for Better Insulation', paragraph 4, Department of the Environment, 1973.
18 'Simple Guidance Notes for those Engaged in Helping Old People', DHSS, September 1972.
19 Letter from the DHSS to Michael Dunne of the Research Institute for Consumer Affairs, 11 November 1976.
20 The words of a DHSS spokesman quoted by Mary Manning in 'Cold Shoulder for the Elderly?', *Community Care*, 2 March 1977.
21 The figures are 92.7%, 1973; 91.7%, 1974; 88.7%, 1975; 96.3% for the third quarter of 1976. See *Housing and Construction Statistics*, No. 20, HMSO, 1977; figures based on tenders approved.
22 For a discussion about 'social costs and social change' *see* R. M. Titmuss, *Social Policy, An Introduction*. George Allen & Unwin, 1974 Chapter 5.

23 According to the 1973 General Household Survey (Great Britain) 32% of older small households had central heating and 25% of individuals aged 60 or over. *General Household Survey,* HMSO, 1976, Table 2.1B.

24 Department of the Environment, Circular 160/74.

25 'The thermal environment. Heat insulation: Whither Research'. Paper to conference on Innovation in the Construction Industry.

26 A. Parker, 'Domestic Heating in Great Britain', *Journal of the Institute of Fuel,* December 1947.

27 *Heating and Ventilation of Dwellings,* op. cit., p. 85.

28 National Consumer Council, *Paying for Fuel,* HMSO, 1976, p. 106.

29 Building Research Establishment, *Energy Conservation: a study of energy consumption in buildings and possible means of saving energy in housing.* A BRE Working Party Report, Department of the Environment, 1975.

30 ibid., para. 4.14.3.

31 ibid., para. 5.2.

32 *Heating and Ventilation of Dwellings,* op. cit., para. 4.3.

33 Department of the Environment, 'Improvement of Older Housing', Circular 160/74, para. 14.

34 *Energy Saving in the Home,* Department of Energy and Central Office of Information, 1975.

35 Department of the Environment, *Housing and Construction Statistics,* (various editions).

36 *Energy Conservation,* op. cit., p. 11.

37 House of Lords Hansard, 16 March 1976. No. 964, Col. 209–10.

38 DHSS *Social Security Statistics,* 1975. HMSO, 1977. Table 34.65.

39 Department of the Environment, Circular 160/74.

40 In its first year of operation local authorities did not submit any applications for these grants.

41 H.C. deb. No. 1083, Col. 1118.

42 Child Poverty Action Group, *Cold Comfort,* 1974.

43 This account of the project is based on 'Experimental Heating Projects for the Elderly', interim report, DOE, Housing Development Directorate, June 1977; and 'Heating Improvements in Old People's Dwellings', Research Institute for Consumer Affairs, 1977, (Draft).

44 For a discussion of the problems of the privately rented housing sector and policy proposals, *see* Malcolm Wicks, *Rented Housing and Social Ownership,* Fabian Society, 1973.

45 For a guide to the extensive literature on this subject *see* A. E. Haseler, *District Heating: An Annotated Bibliography.* Property Services Agency, Library Services. Department of the Environment. Second Edition, 1977.

46 A. E. Haseler, *District Heating–Warmth from Waste.* Institute of Fuel, 1977, p. 2.

47 *District Heating Combined with Electricity Generation in the United Kingdom.* Prepared by the District Heating Working Party of the combined Heat and Power Group. Energy paper No. 20, Department of Energy, HMSO, 1977, Part 2.

48 'No less a person than one of the Brunels is said in "Suggestion for the

Architectural Improvement of the Western Part of London" by Sidney Smirke (1834) to have suggested to the author "the practicability of laying on heat to a long range of these dwellings from a common source, a contrivance, which, if perfected, would be of inestimable importance in London, where the high price of fuel is so great a burthen upon the poor".' Quoted by C. H. Doherty in *Practices in the Domestic Field*. Symposium on Heating and Ventilation for a Human Environment, Institution of Mechanical Engineers, 1967.

49 'District Heating', *Oil and Gas Firing*. February, March and April 1968, p. 1.

50 'District Heating', *Domestic Heating*. Summer 1968, p. 12.

51 Circular 82/71, 'District Heating: A Checklist and Commentary,' November 1971, p. 1.

52 *District Heating combined with electricity generation in the United Kingdom*, op. cit., p. 18.

53 *Housing and Construction Statistics*, No. 18, Table, 31, HMSO, 1976 (figures relate to approved tenders).

54 *District heating combined with electricity generation in the United Kingdom*, op. cit., p. 3.

55 ibid., p. 8.

56 ibid., p. 12.

57 loc. cit.

58 ibid., p. 13.

59 loc. cit. A Building Research Establishment Working Party report concluded that 'there would seem to be grounds for a thorough examination of the potential for combined generation schemes in selected areas of the UK.' *Energy Conservation: a study of energy consumption in buildings and possible means of saving energy in housing*, BRE, DOE, 1975, p. 18.

60 *See* National Consumer Council, *Hypothermia, Appendix 3*, 'Paying for Fuel', HMSO, 1976; Department of Energy, *Review of Payment and Collection Methods for Gas and Electricity Bills*, Report of an informal enquiry (Oakes Report), June 1976; Select Committee on Nationalised Industries, *Gas and Electricity Prices*, House of Commons Paper 353, HMSO, 1976.

61 National Consumer Council, op. cit., p. 2.

62 ibid., pp. 61–2,

63 For a discussion of these issues, *see* Chapter 4 of the National Consumer Council report.

64 *Supplementary Benefits Commission Annual Report*, 1976, para. 12.5.

65 *See* p. 73 of the National Consumer Council report, op. cit., for a brief description of this scheme.

66 National Consumer Council, op. cit., pp. 74–5.

67 ibid., p. 74.

68 *Review of Payment and Collection Methods for Gas and Electricity Bills*, op. cit.

69 *Gas and Electricity Prices*, op. cit.

70 Marigold Johnson and Mark Rowland, *Fuel Debts and the Poor*, Child Poverty Action Group, 1976.

71 British Association of Settlements, 'A Right to Fuel', 1975.

72 *See* HC Deb., Vol. 922, No. 14, columns 478–81, for text of the code 'Payments of Electricity and Gas Bills', and Mr Benn's announcement of its introduction.

73 *See* HC Deb., Vol. 916, No. 516, columns 540–1 for the Secretary of State for Energy's (Mr Benn) announcement of the scheme. *See also* HC Deb, Vol. 919, No. 189, columns 595–6.

74 Ministry of Housing and Local Government, *Council Housing: Purposes, Procedures and Priorities* (Cullingworth Report), HMSO, 1969, para. 289.

75 Department of the Environment, Department of Health and Social Security, Welsh Office, 'Housing for Old People: A Consultation Paper', April 1976, para. 3.1.

76 Department of the Environment, 'English House Condition Survey 1976', Press Notice 321, 28 June 1977.

77 *Council Housing: Purposes, Procedures and Priorities,* op. cit., para. 289.

78 *Housing Statistics, Great Britain,* No. 8, HMSO, 1968, and *Housing and Construction Statistics* (various editions).

79 'Housing for Old People: A Consultation Paper', op. cit., para. 7.

Chapter 10: Social Policy and the Old and Cold

1 K. J. Collins, Caroline Dore, A. N. Exton-Smith, R. H. Fox, I. C. MacDonald and Patricia M. Woodward, 'Accidental hypothermia and impaired temperature homeostasis in the elderly' *British Medical Journal,* 1977, Vol. 1, pp. 353–6.

2 Arlene Goldman, A. N. Exton-Smith, Grace Francis and Ann O'Brien, 'A Pilot Study of Low Body Temperatures in Old People Admitted to Hospital', *Journal of the Royal College of Physicians,* Vol. II, No. 3, April 1977.

3 Office of Population Censuses and Surveys, *The Registrar General's Statistical Review of England and Wales for the Year 1973,* Part 1 (A), Tables, Medical, HMSO, 1975, Table 5.

4 Office of Population Censuses and Surveys, *Population Trends* 1, HMSO, Autumn 1975, Table 29.

5 G. M. Bull and Joan Morton, 'Relationship of Temperature With Death Rates from all Causes and from Certain Respiratory and Arteriosclerotic Diseases in Different Age Groups', *Age and Ageing,* 1975, **4,** 232.

6 Arlene Goldman *et al,* op. cit.

7 Alison Macfarlane, 'Daily Deaths in Greater London', *Population Trends,* 5, HMSO, Autumn 1976, p. 24.

8 Central Policy Review Staff, *A Joint Framework for Social Policies,* HMSO, 1975.

Bibliography

General

British Medical Association, 'Accidental Hypothermia in the Elderly', *British Medical Journal, 1964, 2, 1255.

Exton-Smith, A. N., 'Accidental Hypothermia', *British Medical Journal,* 22 December 1973, 727.

Fox, R. H., Woodward, Patricia M., Fry, A. J., Collins, J. C., and MacDonald, I. C., 'Diagnosis of Accidental Hypothermia of the Elderly', *Lancet,* February 27, 1971, pp 424–427.

Fox, Ronald, *Warmth and the Elderly,* Age Concern, 1974.

Gray, M., Johnson, M., Seagrave, J., and Dunne, M., *A Policy for Warmth,* Fabian Society, 1977.

Green, Michael F., *Hypothermia,* Appendix 3, Paying for Fuel, National Consumer Council, HMSO, 1976.

Maclean, D., and Emslie-Smith, D., *Accidental Hypothermia,* Blackwell Scientific Publications Ltd., 1977.

Taylor, Geoffrey, 'The Problem of Hypothermia in the Elderly', *The Practitioner,* December 1964, Vol. 193.

Medical and Social Surveys

Allen, W. H., 'Accidental Hypothermia in Hertfordshire during the Winters of 1966–7 and 1967–8, *Public Health,* 1969, Vol. 83, 229–239.

Collins, K. J., Dore, Caroline, Exton-Smith, A. N., Fox, R. H., Mac-Donald, I. C., and Woodward, Patricia M., 'Accidental Hypothermia and Impaired Temperature Homeostasis in the Elderly', *British Medical Journal,* 1977, 1, 353.

Fox, R. H., MacGibbon, R., Davies, Louise, Woodward, Patricia M., 'Problem of the Old and Cold', *British Medical Journal,* 6 January 1973.

Fox, R. H., Woodward, Patricia M., Exton-Smith, A. N., Green, M. F., Donnison, D. V., and Wicks, M. H., 'Body Temperatures in the Elderly: A National Study of Physiological, Social and Environmental Conditions', *British Medical Journal,* 27 January 1973.

Goldman, Arlene, Exton-Smith, A. N., Francis, Grace, and O'Brien, Ann, 'A Pilot Study of Low Body Temperatures in Old People Admitted to Hospital', *Journal of the Royal College of Physicians,* 1977, Vol. 11, No. 3.

Harling, Jill and Gullick, Stephen, A Study of Living Conditions Among the Aged in Birmingham, carried out by students of Birmingham University for the Wallace Lawler Friendship Fund, July 1969.

Howitt, L. F., 'Death in Scotland from Malnutrition and/or Hypothermia, 1968', *Health Bulletin, Scottish Home and Health Department,* January 1971, Vol. 29, No. 1.

Islington Task Force, *Old and Cold in Islington . . . A Question of Survival,* Islington Task Force, Islington Poverty Action Group and Islington Consumers' Group, 1971.

Report by the Hypothermia Sub-Committee of the Welfare Group of the Society of Medical Officers of Health, 'A Pilot Survey into the Occurrence of Hypothermia in Elderly People living at home', *Public Health,* 1968, Vol. 32, No. 5.

Royal College of Physicians, *Report of Committee on Accidental Hypothermia,* Royal College of Physicians, 1966.

Task Force, *Left in the Cold,* (prepared by Lilian Fleet), Task Force, (undated).

Williams, B. T., 'Oral Temperatures of Elderly Applicants for Welfare Services', *Gerontologia Clinica,* 1968, 10, 281–287.

Clinical Studies

Duguid, H., Simpson, R. G., and Stowers, J. M., 'Accidental Hypothermia', *Lancet,* 1961, 2, 1213.

Emslie-Smith, D., 'Accidental Hypothermia. A Common Condition with a Pathognomonic Electrocardiogram', *Lancet,* 1958, 2, 492.

McNicol, M. W., and Smith, R., 'Accidental Hypothermia', *British Medical Journal,* 1964, 1, 19.

Prescott, L. F., Peard, Mary C., and Wallace, I. R., 'Accidental Hypothermia. A Common Condition', *British Medical Journal,* 1962, 2, 1367.

Rees, J. R., 'Accidental Hypothermia', *Lancet,* 1958, 1, 556.

Rosin, A. J., and Exton-Smith, A. N., 'Clinical Features of Accidental Hypothermia, with some Observations on Thyroid Function', *British Medical Journal,* 1964, 1, 16.

Appendix

Table A.1

Socio-economic Characteristics of those with 'Low' and 'Normal' Morning Urine Temperatures

No. of Subjects:	'Low' 98 %	'Normal' 699 %	Total: 1020 %	
Sex				
Male	26	41	38	0.005>p
Female	74	59	62	>0.001
Marital Status				
Married	44	50	47	
Single	6	10	10	N.S.
Widowed	49	38	41	
Divorced/Separated	1	2	2	
Age				
65–69	28	40	37	
70–74	30	32	31	
75–79	23	15	17	0.05>p
80–84	11	8	9	>0.02
85+	8	5	6	
Household Composition				
Living alone	40	32	34	N.S.
Not living alone	60	68	66	
Physical Mobility				
'Can get about'	88	93	91	N.S.
'Cannot get about'	12	7	9	
Housing				
Tenure:				
Owner-occupied	31	40	39	
Local authority rented	50	37	38	
Housing association	1	2	3	N.S.
Private rented unfurnished	16	19	19	
Private rented furnished	1	1	1	
Type:				
Detached	8	11	12	
Semi-detached	31	27	27	
Terraced	33	34	33	
Part-house/rooms	5	4	4	N.S.
Flat/Maisonette (purpose built)	19	19	20	
Flat (converted)	—	2	2	
Bed-sit	4	1	2	
Amenities:				
Exclusive use of fixed bath; kitchen sink; W.C. indoors; hot water at sink, bath and hand basin	65	71	70	
Lacking exclusive use of one or more amenity	35	29	30	N.S.
Heating				
With central heating	19	24	23	N.S.
Without central heating	81	76	77	
Supplementary Benefits				
Receiving benefit	50	33	34	p<0.001
Not receiving benefit	49	67	66	

Table A.2

Receipt of Supplementary Pension by
A.M. Living-room and Minimum Bedroom Temperatures

Supplementary Pension	Total	Minimum Bedroom Temperature					A.M. Living-room Temperature				
		<8	8<10	10<12	12<16	16+	0–13	14–15	16–17	18+	Cold A.M. and P.M.
Total:	1,020	136	203	269	251	73	242	274	228	237	56
Yes	34%	29%	37%	30%	32%	37%	31%	38%	33%	32%	29%
No	66%	71%	63%	69%	66%	62%	68%	62%	66%	67%	71%
				N.S.					N.S.		

Table A.3

Weekly Income by A.M. Living-room, Minimum Bedroom
and Urine Temperatures (A.M.)

	Total	Minimum Bedroom Temperature					A.M. Living-room Temperature					Urine Temperature A.M.	
		<8	8<10	10<12	12<16	16+	0–13	14–15	16–17	18+	Cold A.M. and P.M.	35.5 and Under	36.0+
Single Persons Weekly Income													
Total:	538	67	102	145	122	40	134	148	118	112	35	55	353
Up to £7.50	33%	45%	32%	33%	30%	23%	32%	39%	31%	26%	34%	38%	33%
£7.50 – £10.50	38%	34%	34%	33%	39%	55%	36%	38%	37%	43%	40%	42%	39%
More than £10.50	29%	21%	33%	34%	30%	23%	32%	24%	31%	31%	26%	20%	29%
Married Couples Weekly Income													
Total:	482	69	101	124	129	33	108	126	110	125	21	43	346
Up to £12	35%	32%	41%	31%	37%	18%	33%	37%	41%	30%	48%	37%	34%
£12 – £15	27%	26%	26%	31%	23%	27%	27%	24%	20%	33%	33%	33%	26%
More than £15	39%	42%	34%	39%	40%	55%	40%	40%	39%	38%	19%	30%	40%

All categories N.S.

Table A.4

Receipt of Supplementary Benefit, Age, and Urine Temperatures (A.M.)

	All				65–69				70–74				75–79				80–84				85+			
	Low		Normal		Low		Normal		Low		Normal		Low		Normal		Low		Normal		Low		Normal	
	No.	%	No.	%	No.	%	No.	%	No.	%	No.	%	No.	%	No.	%	No.	%	No.	%	No.	%	No.	%
Receiving Benefit	49	50	228	33	11	41	88	31	13	45	70	31	12	52	34	31	7	64	26	47	6	75	10	31
Not Receiving Benefit	48	49	465	67	16	59	191	68	16	55	153	68	11	48	72	67	3	27	29	53	2	25	20	63
Total:	97		693		27		279		29		223		23		106		10		55		8		30	

p<0.001

Table A.5

Night-time Safeguards against the Cold
by Minimum Bedroom Temperatures

| | *Total* | *Minimum Bedroom Temperature* | | | | |
		<8	*8<10*	*10<12*	*12<16*	*16+*
Total	1,020	136	203	269	251	73
Safeguards						
Hot-water bottle	44%	54%	43%	45%	43%	33%
Electric blanket	37%	38%	47%	37%	38%	38%
Extra blankets: Making a total of:—						
1—2	25%	24%	25%	27%	22%	29%
3—4	51%	51%	53%	51%	54%	51%
5—6	9%	9%	9%	12%	7%	3%
Warmer nightwear	50%	54%	52%	49%	50%	41%
Shut all windows	62%	68%	58%	67%	59%	62%

In addition to those noted above, 3 respondents used none of the above 'Safeguards' and 16 mentioned other methods.

Table A.6

Assessment of Subjects' Weight by Room and Body Temperatures

	Total	Minimum Bedroom Temperature					Living-room Temperatures A.M.				Urine Temperature A.M.		
		<8	8<10	10<12	12<16	16+	0–13	14–15	16–17	18+	Cold A.M. and P.M.	Under 35.5	36.0+
Total	1,020	136	203	269	251	73	242	274	228	237	56	98	699
1. Very obese	*%	1%	*%	1%	—	—	*%	1%	—	*%	—	1%	*%
2. Obese	3%	4%	2%	2%	3%	1%	2%	3%	2%	4%	2%	2%	2%
3. Somewhat overweight	23%	22%	29%	24%	20%	27%	22%	26%	23%	22%	21%	24%	23%
4. Normal	55%	61%	51%	54%	61%	52%	56%	53%	59%	55%	63%	47%	59%
5. Somewhat underweight	14%	10%	15%	17%	12%	11%	14%	16%	13%	13%	5%	15%	13%
6. Emaciated	2%	1%	1%	*%	1%	4%	3%	1%	1%	2%	5%	5%	1%
7. Very emaciated	*%	—	—	—	—	1%	—	—	—	1%	—	1%	*%
				N.S.					N.S.			$0.025 > p > 0.01$	

Table A.7

'Comfort Votes' by Temperatures

Table	Question	'Low' / 'Normal'	Living-room Temp. A.M.	Min. Bedroom Temp.
5.4	Ever feel cold indoors	**	**	N.S.
5.5	Hands ever feel numb or cold indoors	*	*	N.S.
5.5	Hand comfort (at interview)	*	**	**
5.6	Body comfort (at interview)	N.S.	**	**
5.7	Preference for warmth	N.S.	**	**
6.9	Would like more heat in house	—	**	*

** p<0.01   * 0.05>p>0.01   N.S. = Not significant

Table A.8

Percentage of Persons Living Alone by Activities the Previous Day; 1962$^\phi$ and 1972

	1962	1972
Activities		
Listening to radio	63	69
Watching television	37	77
Going for walk	41	50
Shopping	40	51
Having visitors	42	57
Visiting friends*	27	30
Meeting friends somewhere†	26	43
None of these things	2	—
Went to work	—	3

ø By way of comparison with the 1972 survey results, the table includes the responses given to very similar questions asked in the 1962 survey reported in: Shanas, Townsend *et al, Old People in Three Industrial Societies*, Routledge & Kegan Paul, 1968, Table ix–4.
* The 1972 survey enquired about visiting friends/*relatives*
† The 1972 survey enquired about meeting friends outside home

Table A.9

Sex, Marital Status and Household Composition by A.M. Living-room and Minimum Bedroom Temperatures

	Total	Minimum Bedroom Temperatures					A.M. Living-room Temperatures				Cold A.M. and P.M.
		<8	8<10	10<12	12<16	16+	0–13	14–15	16–17	18+	
	1,020	136	203	269	251	73	242	274	228	237	56
Total											
Sex											
Male	38%	40%	43%	37%	38%	36%	44%	38%	32%	41%	36%
Female	62%	60%	57%	63%	62%	64%	56%	62%	68%	59%	64%
Marital Status											
1. Married	47%	51%	50%	46%	51%	45%	45%	46%	48%	53%	38%
2. Single	10%	9%	12%	8%	7%	8%	16%	10%	6%	8%	20%
3. Widowed	41%	39%	36%	45%	41%	44%	38%	43%	45%	37%	39%
4. Divorced/Separated	2%	1%	2%	1%	1%	3%	2%	1%	1%	3%	4%
Houshold Composition											
Living Alone	34%	32%	31%	32%	28%	41%	38%	35%	31%	27%	39%
Not Living Alone	66%	68%	69%	68%	72%	59%	62%	65%	69%	73%	61%

0.25>p>0.01 for marital status by A.M. living-room. All other results not significant.

Table A.10

Age by Minimum Bedroom and A.M. Living-room Temperatures

	Total	Minimum Bedroom Temperatures					A.M. Living-room Temperatures				
		<8	8<10	10<12	12<16	16+	0–13	14–15	16–17	18+	Cold A.M. and P.M.
Total	1,020	136	203	269	251	73	242	274	228	237	56
Age											
65–69	37%	37%	40%	40%	33%	37%	38%	39%	36%	34%	38%
70–74	31%	32%	36%	29%	29%	33%	28%	31%	31%	35%	39%
75–79	17%	18%	13%	18%	20%	14%	18%	16%	17%	18%	9%
80–84	9%	6%	7%	9%	11%	7%	10%	9%	9%	7%	11%
85+	6%	7%	3%	4%	7%	10%	7%	4%	7%	6%	4%

Table A.11

Number of Bedrooms and Use of Bedrooms
by Morning Living-room Temperatures

		A.M. Living-room Temperatures				Cold A.M. and P.M.
	Total	0–13	14–15	16–17	18+	
Total	1,020	242	274	228	237	56
Number of Bedrooms*						
1	19%	16%	16%	18%	22%	18%
2	34%	38%	32%	34%	37%	41%
3	36%	36%	42%	38%	28%	34%
4	5%	6%	5%	5%	5%	5%
5	1%	*%	1%	*%	1%	—
None	5%	4%	4%	4%	7%	2%
Any Bedroom Seldom or Never Used						
Yes	48%	52%	55%	47%	38%	50%
No	52%	48%	45%	53%	62%	50%

p<0.001

* In addition some respondents lived in bed-sits and they are not included in this Table. Their room temperatures are shown in Table 6.3.

Table A.12

Physical Mobility by Living-room Temperatures

		A.M. Living-room Temperatures				Cold A.M. and P.M.
	Total	0–13	14–15	16–17	18+	
Total	1,020	242	274	228	237	56
Respondent Stated that He/She:						
Can get about	91%	90%	90%	95%	89%	95%
Cannot get about	9%	10%	10%	5%	11%	5%

Index